Cover design by Sadie E. Nezich of Concord Consulting, LLC
Editing by Ashley Wiederhold of Grammar Chic, Inc.
Editing and formatting by Amanda E. Clark of Grammar Chic, Inc. -
www.grammarchic.net

ISBN 978-1-4507-2860-7

Published by EDGE Publishing Company
8939 Sweetbriar St.
Manassas, VA 20110
(703)447-3780
www.edgepublishingcompany.com

Praise for

CURING CHRONIC FIBROMYALGIA

**Patrick D. Goonan Top Reviewer on Amazon.com,
MA Psychology—Personal Growth Coach**

Curing Chronic Fibromyalgia – Choosing What Works by author Valerie Lumley, A Unique, Readable, Personal Journey and Roadmap for Victims and Their Families.

I have a unique background both personally and professionally. I started my career as a research scientist and later became committed to working in the field of psychology. In my capacity as a personal growth coach, I have worked with people with chronic illnesses, organizations committed to helping individuals with these diseases and I have suffered from serious illness myself (more than once). In my case, the illness was different, but the sense of helplessness, being alone and frustration with where we are in terms of understanding and dealing with these types of complex multi-system disorders is common ground that I share.

It was certainly a pleasure to review this well-researched, intimate and extremely thorough exploration of options available for those suffering from this devastating disease. The fact that it also chronicles one person's road to recovery is a significant added value. The vulnerability with which the author shares her experiences helps to establish credibility and an atmosphere of compassion and hope. This is capped off by a keen intellect and ability to understand, explain and hold multiple perspectives.

It is from this psychological space that I have reviewed this book. My first observation is that many debilitating illnesses tend to defy a simple reduction to one or a few causes and even deep analysis via the scientific method. I don't think it's a secret to anyone that it is very difficult to predict outcomes in multivariable systems and you only need to tune into the weather or world politics to see numerous examples of our failure to see important connections and emergent qualities within chaotic systems e.g. the brain and nervous system. On the other hand, science is acknowledging this slowly, but perhaps not quickly enough to help many people in need. Chaos and Systems Theories would be examples of manifestations of this significant forward movement. It also appears in such mainstream best–sellers such as the [[ASIN:0345506529 The Love Response: Your Prescription to Turn Off Fear, Anger, and Anxiety to Achieve Vibrant Health and Transform Your Life]], [[ASIN:006251606X The HeartMath Solution: The Institute of HeartMath's Revolutionary Program for Engaging the Power of the Heart's Intelligence]] or [[ASIN:0345490118 Healthy at 100: The Scientifically Proven Secrets of the World's Healthiest and Longest-Lived Peoples]]. In the must read category, I would also include [[ASIN:1883536170 The Healing Brain: Breakthrough Discoveries About How the Brain Keeps Us

Healthy]] and [[ASIN:0805073698 Why Zebras Don't Get Ulcers, Third Edition]] and [[ASIN:039370470X The Mindful Brain: Reflection and Attunement in the Cultivation of Well-Being]].

So, what is an individual person suffering from a serious illness to do? You could place yourself totally into the hands of the medical profession. Certainly, their efforts and achievements have resulted in a life expectancy that people would not have imagined even 100 years ago. However, clearly they don't have all the answers. As I see it, a holistic systems approach is needed that leverages the best that medicine has to offer as well as the extensive experiential information available from individuals who have traveled this road themselves, the various wisdom traditions informed by common sense and better attunement to the body itself. Sometimes, we are too "in our heads" to take the time to do this, but "physician heal thyself," certainly is a quote that seems to ring true and merit considerable attention.

We are fortunate to live during a period where there is a cross fertilization of knowledge, ideas and cultural wisdom. Valerie Lumley has done her homework and provided those suffering from Chronic Fibromyalgia the pluses and minuses of various alternative approaches as well as an in-depth inquiry into her own journey overcoming this disease. I have met her in person and she is healthy, vibrant, youthful and certainly passionate about life. In sense, this book is a also a meta-study or collection of the best of the best information available across disciplines.

I can write much more about the book, but I think the author unconsciously gave her own best testimony when in a recent discussion she nonchalantly said, "I know this illness from the inside out like no other author on the subject. FMS is a very dark tunnel and its victims get lost in despair. I want to stand at the end of this tunnel with bells and whistles and shine a light bright enough for all to see and show them how to guide themselves back to life again. This is my mission." My sense of her was that she embodies this mission and her book bears testimony to this commitment. It is the best book I know of on this subject and she packs a lot of useful material into less than 300 pages. It is my sincere desire that it provides hope for those who are feeling lost in the middle of a desert without a good road map.

After finishing Valerie's book, I would also consider reading [[ASIN:034549802X 8 Weeks to Optimum Health: A Proven Program for Taking Full Advantage of Your Body's Natural Healing Power]], [[ASIN:1590304675 Integral Life Practice: A 21st-Century Blueprint for Physical Health, Emotional Balance, Mental Clarity, and Spiritual Awakening]] and [[ASIN:159120190X Integral Health: The Path to Human Flourishing]]. With that said, I believe one of the most valuable resources is your own body, a way to stay close to it such as a body journal and perhaps the consideration of a new paradigm like the one presented in [[ASIN:0465056741 Philosophy in the Flesh : The Embodied Mind and Its Challenge to Western Thought]]. Independent of any specific belief system you are committed to, I also recommend [[ASIN:1572246952 Buddha's Brain: The Practical Neuroscience of Happiness, Love, and Wisdom]] and [[ASIN:0307407802 Joyful Wisdom: Embracing Change and Finding Freedom]].

Patrick D. Goonan, MA Psychology—Personal Growth Coach

International Chiropractic Association (ICA)
Dr. George Curry, D.C.

"Valerie has cracked the code for chronic fibromyalgia and discovered techniques to release the body's true healing potential."

"This book is a must read for CFS patients to discover the hidden secrets of upper cervical care."

"This book is a comprehensive guide to effective alternatives to traditional drugs for the correction of chronic fibromyalgia ....thank you Valerie!

George B. Curry, D.C. FICA LCP
International Chiropractors Association
Board of Directors
Director of East Coast ICA Division

American Association of Acupuncture and Oriental Medicine
Dr. Doug Newton

Valerie,

Your book is a very thorough and important work and written very carefully!

Dr. Doug Newton – Director of Operations AAAOM
American Association of Acupuncture And Oriental Medicine

International Chiropractic Association (ICA)
Dr. Gene Crestsinger, D.C.

Valerie,
I finished reading your book CURING CHRONIC FIBROMYALGIA last evening. It is a thorough excellent resource for anyone with the symptoms of fibromyalgia that offers hope and remedy for the condition. Thank you for writing this story so others can find a cure as well.

Gene Cretsinger, D.C.
Board Member of the International Chiropractic Association
Cedar Rapids, IA

Oregon Health & Science University (OHSU)
Fibromyalgia Information Foundation
Dr. Robert Bennett, PhD

Dear Valerie,

First the clarity and level of expression is really excellent (did you do much writing in your previous life?)

I always like appropriate quotations and this book did not disappoint.

The "psychological" chapters were really very well done, and I think you got across the philosophy of dealing with chronic pain in a practical and understanding manner.

I liked your section on Dr. St. Amand and Guaifenesin, which was well balanced. We did a whole year's study on Guaifenesin and found that it "worked" but no better than the placebo. See: http://www.myalgia.com/guaif2.htm.

In patients developing FM after a neck injury (typically whiplash in my experience), atlas subluxations and at other levels of the cervical spine should always be considered and treated conservatively – that includes chiropractic manipulation. I agree that the little known aspects of anatomy, such as atrophy of the rectus capitis posterior minor may be relevant to some cases of chronic neck pain (but is yet to be recognized by many pain doctors), but whether the atrophy is the cause or the effect is not yet clear. A friend and colleague of mine from Denmark has published an interesting study of this association: http://www.ncbi.nlm.nih.gov/pubmed/18174844.

The use of various vitamins, nutrients and minerals is a difficult subject. However, I must admit that I personally take many of same supplements that you use! There is increasing evidence that many people have suboptimal levels of vitamin D and the daily recommendation has now gone from 400 IU to 1.000 IU. I obviously have my own set of misperceptions that I have taught myself to set aside when writing.

Katie Holton has some good evidence that some additives such as glutamate and aspartate can aggravate FM symptoms, and we hope to follow that up with a larger study. Katie's study is only the second double blind controlled trial of dietary manipulation in FM; this is sobering when one looks at all the claims on the Internet about food and FM.

Lastly I would draw your attention to an important new development in the understanding of FM tender points and myofascial trigger points. I have always thought they were probably the same, and have mentioned this belief in several manuscripts, but was too lazy to do the experiments. Now there is good evidence that most FM tender points are in fact myofascial trigger points and are major myofascial trigger points are important pain generators, will in my opinion, play an increasingly important role in the effective management of FM. Indeed the role of peripheral pain generators (such as spinal subluxations, infections, dietary excitoxins, persistent stressors etc.) as initiators and maintainers of central sensitization provide a useful paradigm for the current understanding of FM.

My best wishes for a successful book and hopefully an update!

Kind regards,

Dr. Robert Bennett, PhD
Oregon Health & Science University
Fibromyalgia Information Foundation

National Upper Cervical Chiropractic Association (NUCCA)
Steven MacDonald, D.C.

Dear Valerie,

Valerie Lumley's excellent book "Curing Chronic Fibromyalgia, Choosing what Works," is her story of her journey to curing her Fibromyalgia. It is a balanced well thought out holistic approach. It includes the recounting of injuries to her head and neck that began the symptoms of Fibromyalgia and what she had to go through to eventually heal those injuries. She has done an exhaustive study into the effects of these injuries and the damage it did to the balance of her body and the health of her central nervous system. She explains clearly the process that a Patient with Fibromyalgia symptoms needs to explore. Valerie specifically informs that one needs to seek out an Upper Cervical Chiropractic specialist to professionally correct their Head and Neck imbalances that are causing brainstem injuries from injuries to this area. That this is the source of their symptoms. As a specialist in Upper Cervical Chiropractic, who has treated these injuries for 31 years, I can't emphasize enough the importance of properly treating these injuries. The benefits are too great not to ignore. Valerie Lumley has written this book to assist the Fibromyalgia sufferer to insure that they are on the right healing path.

Warm Regards,

Steven N MacDonald, D.C.
Board Certified in the National Upper Cervical Chiropractic Technique
(NUCCA) Member of the NUCCA Board of Directors
Pacific Grove, California

Published by EDGE Publishing Company
Manassas, VA
www.edgepublishingcompany.com

Curing Chronic Fibromyalgia

Valerie Lumley

EDGE Publishing Company
Manassas, VA
www.edgepublishingcompany.com

Table of Contents

Dedication

I want to dedicate this book to my husband, Ron. When we met, I had been highly disillusioned by a previous marriage. This turned out to be a blessing. Not only because illusions are an unhealthy basis for any relationship, if I had not been divorced, I would not have met Ron.

The love and safety I found with Ron helped me learn to be an alchemist, and convert the base metals of daily life into gold. I also learned to be a loving stepmother to his three wonderful children. This became a great adventure, and taught me that the human heart has an infinite capacity for love. Life became something that had a true meaning and purpose for each and every one of us.

They say when you are loved, the soul takes on the task of healing dormant wounds from the past as they begin to surface and expose themselves to the healing powers of love's panacea. Four years after we were married I injured my back and neck, which triggered chronic fibromyalgia syndrome (FMS).

The next 10 years became the turning point in my life when I would begin to enter into what St. John from the 16th century called "The dark night of the soul" or the "cocoon of metamorphosis" where I would eventually emerge and take flight in my truest form.

Through all the FMS years, if not for Ron's love, devotion, and protection, I surely would have resigned and died before my years of a thousand, horrible deaths, and this book and my return to life would not have been possible.

I further dedicate this book to all the fibromyalgia sufferers around the world. Knowing they are suffering needlessly gave me the strength to write this book, and I wish them all success on their journey back to health and in taking their life back from this horrible disease. I also owe a special thanks to everyone who helped in its preparation.

Foreword

Valerie Lumley has quite an amazing story to tell. This book certainly has a higher purpose, as Valerie wrote it with an underlying passion to share her success at curing her illness and to help thousands of people break free from the shackles of their Fibromyalgia.

Valerie came into my office for help in 2008 and made an unforgettable impression. I completed my chiropractic exam, took x-rays of her spine, then told her I would review her findings and explain the results to her on our next visit. Valerie then said to me, "Dr. Ruiz, before our next visit I would like for you to watch a video I have about my condition." I had never had this happen before in my 24 years of practice.

The video was of Valerie giving an explanation about the central nervous system and how the effects of a misaligned first spinal bone in the neck had detrimental effects on her health. I was impressed by her dedication to research on all that she needed to do to become vibrant and healthy again. Valerie asked if I would adjust the subluxation at her C1 and be part of her health team. I of course was happy to have such a knowledgeable, driven and inspirational patient.

Valerie has written a book that shares how Fibromyalgia devastated her health and what she did to regain her life. There are valuable lessons to be learned from Valerie Lumley's life changing story.

~Peter A. Ruiz, D.C.

Foreword

When Valerie Lumley first presented herself at my office in October of 2001 she was quite ill. She had been in bed for the larger part of eight years and explained that she was very weak and that her muscles ached and episodically produced horrific spasms. In spite of this pain, the beautiful woman who sat before me was poised and composed and spoke with great depth and clarity.

On the third visit after four months of treatment Valerie came to the office and said she had a surprise for me. She carried in her guitar case and proceeded to bring out her instrument, saying that she was just going to sing a little song that she had written. She strummed the strings with assurance, but the biggest surprise was her voice. Strong and rich with vibrato, her voice filled the room and literally caused the window panes to shutter in their sills. Her voice was so powerful that I fleetingly worried that the little house that is my office might collapse from the energy.

The pathway of Valerie's journey back to health and the regaining of her vitality is chronicled in this book. The route was circuitous and not without drawbacks. In order to regain her well-being, Valerie sought and found help in the realm of alternative medicine. The integrated approach addresses distress in the physical body with understanding of the nature of disease and its relationship to the mental, emotional and spiritual spheres. As she wound her way out of the labyrinth of fibromyalgia, Valerie found she must also excavate the events of her past, reexamining all that she knew about her early life and illuminating the events with new understanding.

With courage and tenacity Valerie took the initial small and exhausting steps and eventually was able to break free. She learned to trust herself and was able to transform her illness into a sojourn to the core of her true self. What emerged was an inspiring road map for others on the same odyssey.

~Karen Cohen, D.C. CCH

Introduction

Albert Einstein said, "The only true source of knowledge is experience." As a recovered fibromyalgia sufferer who has been well for over three years, I know this condition is curable. He also said, "Imagination is more important than knowledge." People suffering from Chronic Fibromyalgia Syndrome (FMS) are lost in a dark tunnel of despair with no hope from the medical profession of ever getting well. While writing this book, I imagined myself standing at the end of this tunnel shining a light bright enough for all to see, showing them how to guide themselves back out into life again.

My goal in writing this book is to create a paradigm shift in the way FMS is viewed showing it is curable. I have drawn a clear roadmap showing the tens of millions of FMS sufferers worldwide how they can choose to take charge of their condition and take back their life. This being my mission, I am sharing my protocol for a lasting cure that has worked for me and is maintainable and real, after researching and writing this book over 10 years.

I see everything in life as a choice, whether it is an action, inaction, reaction, or a thoughtful response to a person or situation. The choices a person with FMS makes concerning their condition will either make them better or worse. This can be a polarizing responsibility if there is no guideline to follow and the medical profession says taking multiple drugs to manage symptoms is your only option. Then there is also year after year of failed hope that causes an FMS sufferer to give up hoping all together. This book restores hope by providing a comprehensive understanding of FMS and a guideline from which to begin the journey of healing this horrible, devastating disorder.

In 1993, FMS came suddenly into my life like a thief in the night, and made off with my hopes, my dreams, and my future. I was eventually told by the medical profession that "chronic FMS is an incurable, degenerative disease with no known cause or cure, and that all I could do was manage its symptoms with lots of drugs for the rest of my life." I then found myself faced with the most important choice ever: choosing to reject this fate, and commit to healing myself of this supposed incurable syndrome, and take back my life.

I ultimately chose to leave the care of the medical profession that offered me no hope or understanding, and took charge of my condition. I chose to study hard, use myself as a case study, and do everything necessary to succeed. I became relentlessly committed to defeating doubt, making hard and necessary changes, continue learning all I could and apply what I learned, and be tenaciously true to myself. Most importantly, I chose to listen to my innate, instinctive intelligence and rely upon it to guide me.

Chronic disease is an adverse detour off the beaten path that sets a person apart from themselves and apart from others. FMS is an experience full of forced learning, hard choices, and unexpected truths taught by an imposed teacher to a reluctant student. A student who has the power to respond in a myriad of different ways to what they are being taught.

I believe within us we all have surprising capability to use our power of choice. This book chronicles my journey of how I took charge of my condition and became well again after having been bed-ridden with FMS for 2 years and housebound for 10. I want my story to inspire others to respond to this brutal taskmaster in a way that defeats failed hope, moves them forward, and motivates them not to give up on their journey back to health.

Bruce Lee said, "Learning is not enough. We must apply." His wife Linda Lee shared his wisdom with the world. By applying all I have learned to healing this illness, and after four years of following my protocol for a lasting cure using natural, alternative methods that avoid a life-long dependency on drugs with no hope of improvement, I became well again and have maintained the cure for over three years. In many ways at age 61, I am healthier now than ever before in my life.

In this book I speak strictly from experience that has been educated, and not an education that has never been experienced. This experience, along with universal spiritual, moral, and psychological truths, and the support of scientific published research, is the basis for all that I write. What I convey comes from having lived the very things I talk about. Experience and self-education are my credits and qualifications. My success is my degree. Albert Einstein also said, "All knowledge should be converted into action." This moral truth is exactly the force that has compelled me to write this book. With God's guiding hand, I accepted the challenge with faith and optimism.

Preface

This book is a journey into curing chronic fibromyalgia syndrome. I wrote it to provide enlightenment and hope for all who suffer from this horrific illness, to show how to cure it both physically and psychologically. This is the story of how I found my own truth, my struggle to understand and accept it, and how I became secure enough within myself to be my own guide in discovering the cause and the cure of chronic FMS. By developing a realistic perception of myself and others, according to current physical, psychological, and spiritual truths, I was able to achieve this goal.

William Shakespeare wrote in Hamlet, "This above all, to thyne own self be true, and as the night follows the day, thou then canst not be false to any man." This, among other wonderful quotes from Henry Thoreau, Rudyard Kipling, Bruce Lee, Albert Einstein, Buddha, Jesus, and a wide variety of modern day thinkers, has provided me with support and encouragement. I hope you will feel the same way.

Albert Einstein said, "Great spirits have always encountered violent opposition from mediocre minds." I believe that our resistance to change is at the root of the human inertia that prevents us from moving out of our current position, and into a new and better one, possibly leaving us stuck where we are. Surely the purpose of our life is not to choose to live stuck in one place. I believe the purpose for our life is simply to find our own truth and believe in it, to learn how to balance being both mortal and spiritual beings, and to apply what we learn to our lives so that we can continue to move forward as we evolve into more loving human beings.

If we utilize the capacity of our individual gifts to their fullest extent, we have the potential of making a valuable contribution to the world. These kinds of achievements honor the precious life we have been given. My greatest hope is to inspire others to courageously scout out and forge a new trail for themselves that will free them from chronic FMS, and lead them to a state of physical, psychological, emotional, and spiritual health and well being. Now this, I believe, is worth the effort!

The Term God

The term God, as I use it in this book, does not represent a specific religion or sect per se. The term God as I use it represents:

The creator of all that is and is not created.
The giver of all that is and is not given.
The taker of all that is and is not taken.
The knower of all that is and is not known.
The seer of all that is and is not seen.
The teacher of all that is and is not taught.
The all-merciful forgiver of all there is to forgive.
The embodiment of all that is and is not real.
The presence of all that is and is not now.
The possessor of all that is past and all that is yet to come.
The keeper of all that is and is not sacred.
The preserver of life everlasting.
The body of love eternal.
The one who is the one.
The one who is in us all.
The one who is all.

These Are My Wishes For You

"May you always feel loved. May you find serenity and tranquility in a world you may not always understand. May the pain you have known and the conflict you have experienced give you the strength to walk through life facing each new situation with courage and optimism. Always know that there are those whose love and understanding will always be there, even when you feel most alone. May you discover enough goodness in others to believe in a world of peace. May a kind word, a reassuring touch, and a warm smile be yours every day of your life, and may you give these gifts as well as receive them. Remember the sunshine when the storm seems unending. Teach love to those who know hate, and let that love embrace you as you go into the world. May the teachings of those you admire become part of you, so that you may call upon them. Remember, those whose lives you have touched and who have touched yours are always a part of you, even if the encounters were less than you would have wished. It is the content of the encounter that is more important than its form. May you not become too concerned with material matters, but instead place immeasurable value on the goodness in your heart. Find time in each day to see beauty and love in the world around you. Realize that each person has limitless abilities, but each of us is different in our own way. What you may feel you lack in one regard may be more than compensated for in another. What you feel you lack in the present may become one of your strengths in the future. May you see your future as one filled with promise and possibility. Learn to view everything as a worthwhile experience. May you find enough inner strength to determine your own worth by yourself, and not be dependent on another's judgment of your accomplishments. May you always be loved."

Sandra Sturtz Hauss

Chapter One
Distancing Dysfunctional Relationships

The pathway to healing begins with detachment

Dysfunctional relationships are exhausting and stressful, and so is chronic fibromyalgia syndrome (FMS). First and foremost, FMS is a condition that is exacerbated by stress and combining dysfunctional relationships with FMS it is a recipe for disaster. The stress of FMS alone is nearly beyond what words can describe. I remember a time when my brain was receiving more pain signals than it could process, so many that my mind could not even form sentences, and if it could I was too weak to utter them. A time when my muscles were so tight all over I could not bend or turn my head without injuring myself or pulling out a rib, and all the muscles in my body felt as though they were laced with ground glass. A time when I was on fire with burning skin, buzzing with bio-chemical overcharge, too weak to cry out and afraid to cry because it would worsen my pain. Noise was torture, being touched was torture, pain had become everything and everything had become pain. I needed major assistance and all I could do was lie in bed and not move. I was completely caught in a vise of excruciating non-stop agony, the likes of which I had never imagined possible.

When I forced my mind to think and tried to grasp what I was experiencing, I thought, "Why am I not unconscious from all this pain? How can I go on enduring this hellish non-life 24/7 for the rest of my days?" I knew there was no way in heaven I could do this, and no way in hell I was going to accept it as my fate. Somewhere in all this hopelessness, depression, and purgatory, my spirit rose up and chose to conquer this living nightmare into which I was dispatched and free myself from chronic fibromyalgia syndrome. No matter what it took, I was going to prevail.

Finding a place to begin required recognizing where the disease lived: the central nervous system. This was my beginning. This was when I realized I had to eliminate all the stress in my life I could. This meant identifying the major stressors and making some major changes and hard decisions. The starting place became distancing myself from the dysfunctional people in my life with as much love, forgiveness, and compassion as possible at the time. The stress of these relationships was worsening my condition, and I was forced to protect myself. I had to learn to understand the stress these relationships caused, and what the dysfunction was, in order to be at peace with my decision and continue my quest for a cure.

Dysfunctional relationships are typically wrought with crises and drama, and there are many clinical descriptions that identify the various aspects of dysfunction. However, a simple way to describe dysfunction is emotional and psychological immaturity and an inability to maintain healthy boundaries and appropriate behavior. Participants in dysfunctional relationships are often codependent on each other.

A good therapist helped me educate myself and discover that I no longer had to struggle in my relationships with dysfunctional people and that I had every right to live my life apart from them. Freeing myself of entanglements with dysfunctional people enabled me to leave the past behind with forgiveness, compassion, and loving detachment. Before arriving at this point, my desires to be healthy were simply hands reaching beyond their grasp.

Cutting the Ties

Nelson Mandela said, "Judging without understanding in order to serve your own feelings is selfish thinking." When I first cut ties with the dysfunctional people in my life, I experienced a variety of reactions from those I chose to distance myself from, such as: lack of respect, anger, lack of boundaries, and intrusiveness. While loving, healthy individuals will exhibit similar behavior when faced with a separation from someone they care for, the reactions I experienced were far from healthy. In therapy, I learned the difference between the kind of anger shown by a healthy individual and that which has been altered by dysfunction. I also learned that the responses I experienced are common, predictable, and even natural in dysfunctional relationships.

My FMS was triggered by an exercise injury to my neck and back, which compounded an old neck injury. Suddenly, the psychological stress caused by the dysfunction in my life became a major exacerbation to my condition. One of my physicians advised that unless I distanced myself from the dysfunction I would have no chance of recovery. It became clear that fibromyalgia would not allow me to further tolerate any more of this kind of stress.

The disease began to take over my life. It forced me to seek help and educate myself about the complexity of dysfunctional relationships and to see others as they really are. Through this understanding, I acquired the compassion I needed to authentically forgive others for their failings, and the strength to detach from them emotionally. I now understood that, in taking responsibility for myself, I did not have to take responsibility for others.

Stay the Course

Second Timothy 4:7-8 says, "I have fought a good fight, I have finished my course, I have kept the faith, henceforth there is laid up for me a crown of righteousness, which the Lord, the righteous judge, shall give me at the day, but not to me only, but unto all them also that love his appearing." Because I worked so hard to achieve complete understanding, compassion, and forgiveness while eliminating the most stressful parts of my life, I now experience inner peace of mind.

I try to honor myself (one of the seven sacred truths that correspond with the seven Chakras of Hindu Kundalini), stand for health, safety, detached compassion, and forgiveness, appropriate tolerance and, most of all, love. Part of the healing process is letting go of anger, both with others and with yourself. I am no longer angry with those who have caused me harm in the past, and I am not angry with myself for choosing my health over their feelings. Given the choice between healing yourself from chronic FMS or coping with dysfunction, it is natural to choose yourself. Because stress exacerbates FMS, the pathway to healing may begin with detaching from dysfunctional relationships for as long as you need to get well. Making this choice allowed me to eliminate major stressors in my life; without this additional stress, and the extra pain it caused, my central nervous system finally had a chance to heal.

Having learned to understand the importance of being true to myself, defining myself by my boundaries, and detaching from those incapable of respecting them, I became free to concentrate on the physical part of my healing process with great success and am now mentally and physically healthier than I have ever been. It has been a difficult journey, but it has been well worth it. In spite of all the pain, I enjoy the experience of learning and growing and applying what I learn to my life. I simply had to learn to develop a new, more informed view of my relationships and myself and abandon the old one. "Grin and bear it" no longer worked for me.

Adjust Your Point Of View

To take charge of your life and condition, you may have to adjust your point of view about love and relationships. F. Scott Peck, author of *Peo-*

ple of the Lie, referred to love as an act of will: a choice to extend one-self for the sake and betterment of another. I agree with him whole-heartedly. Conversely, guilt, false obligation, and misplaced responsibility bind us emotionally and psychologically to dysfunctional relationships. Our biological parents are the vehicles that brought us into this world. They may or may not fully understand the privilege of caring for and nurturing one of God's creations, but they would have done the best they could with what they had at the time, no matter who their children were. For better or for worse, their parenting skills and capacities for nurturing and love were engrained in them long before their children were born, and had nothing whatsoever to do with you. Children of dys-functional parents are simply not responsible for their parent's morals, personal standards, strengths, or weaknesses.

Furthermore, I believe that, regardless of who your family is, what you learn by experiencing them is invaluable. Life's lessons come to us from a variety of sources. Pragmatically speaking, our biological family can be seen simply as one of these sources, whether they are dysfunction-al or not. What we learn from them, good or bad, becomes an important part of how we experience our lives and the way we choose to see our own reality.

Finally, all our relationships can be seen as stepping-stones on the path to enlightenment, self-realization, and fulfillment, rather than as de-termining factors to our life's success. With this perspective, we can see them not as an end, but as a valuable means toward our spiritual evolution. Our lives are not meant to be stagnate microcosms defined by peo-ple or value systems; our lives are meant to be like the ever-expanding universe, moving outward and away from the previous positions of the past. Like the universe, we can expand outward into new endeavors and healthier relationships. Unlike the stars in the universe, which are forever grouped together within solar systems and galaxies, we can choose who surrounds us on our outward path.

When we feel our life force being sucked into a black hole by the gravity of false obligations and misplaced responsibilities, we can choose to pull away and redirect our course. We can move to different places and see things from different points of view. Like the universe, our lives are full of never-ending possibilities and wonders beyond our imagina-tion. Our lives are bigger than what took place in our past or what is hap-pening today. In the end, we are the sum total of our choices. Like the stars in our wondrous and mysterious universe, these choices are endless. My father once said, "It's not how you start out but how you end up that counts."

Embrace the Mysterious

Albert Einstein said, "The most beautiful thing we can experience is the mysterious." To me one of the great mysteries in the universe is love. Where does love come from, why are we so compelled to have it within us, and why do we need it for our very survival? The answer to these questions I believe has to do with the nature of the human spirit and its eternal connection to its creator. "God is love" is a well-known spiritual concept that is widely accepted throughout the world. Perhaps, as human beings who are physically separated from our creator, we simply require a continuous connection to God in order to maintain a balance between our spiritual being and the physical realm into which we were born. Love serves as this vital connection. Without it, we are out of balance, vulnerable, and lost in darkness.

John Grey, author of *Men are from Mars – Women are From Venus,* said, "When you can't get what you need from one source, and all you are getting is pain and disappointment, then stop looking there, and turn away and look somewhere else." I agree with him. When a relationship is incapable of providing you what you need, find another source, find someone else who is capable of being a healthy and nurturing source of love.

Your soul needs love and nurturing, and it does not matter who provides it. A "parent or family of choice" can provide the sense of healthy unity and caring respect that you may not be able to find within your own biological family. Furthermore, a biological connection does not constitute a reason to maintain close ties, especially if that connection is an unhealthy and destructive drain on your energy. In the bigger picture, family labels have no value.

Discard the Labels

As we mature, the labels of those around us no longer matter and it is up to us, not labels, to determine who will help us achieve success. Family labels, conditioning to duty, false obligations, misplaced responsibility, illegitimate guilt, and fear are all unhealthy shackles that can enslave the soul and prevent it from expansion and fulfillment. Although it may be difficult, it is possible to develop a detached form of compassion and love for others while remaining distant from them. This is an important part of detaching from dysfunctional people in your life.

I call this "living in loving detachment" and it has become my personal motto. This detached form of compassion and love can simply come from learning to appreciate a shared sense of spiritual creation and physical mortality, and not from the psychological enslavement of co-dependency where responsibility is reversed. You are only responsible for yourself.

The most important choice you make in this life is to UN-enslave your spirit through compassionate forgiveness and loving detachment, freeing your spirit to soar into the unknown with courage and faith in yourself. The title of Susan Jeffers' book, *Feel the Fear and Do It Anyway,* sums up the very essence of courage. It is not courage if there exists no fear.

Fear causes us to be careful, alert, and to pay attention to what is presented to us. In this way as long as you remain in the present, fear is a loyal friend. Embrace your fear and follow through with what you truly need for yourself, rather than live with the underlying fear of being too helpless to take charge of your own life. Growing up is a choice like all others, and the cost of making wise and sometimes painful choices in your healing interest is a small fraction of the cost of choosing to be stuck in the same place for the rest of your life.

Albert Einstein also said, "We cannot solve problems by using the same kind of thinking we used when we created them." Detaching from dysfunctional relationships and cutting the ties that bind you to them can be as simple as choosing to think in healthier terms, terms that put you in charge of yourself, your life, and your condition. Albert Einstein is also famous for his simple words, "Think differently!" See the man on the moon as the profile of someone new and different, instead of the same old face. See your partial or non-participation in a dysfunctional relationship as a choice for your own betterment.

Stop Being a Team Player

Dysfunctional relationships sap your life-force energy. They require building protective walls that take energy to maintain. The enormous amount of energy required to maintain these walls barely leaves you enough energy to live your own life, and comes at the expense of your health and personal growth. This outlay in energy is also extremely detrimental to healing chronic FMS.

To truly heal your illness and regain your mental and physical and psychological health, you need every bit of energy you can produce. Chronic energy deficit is a part of FMS. You cannot afford to be exposed to unnecessary outside stressors that are beyond your control. Outside stress causes serious pain, flare-ups and exacerbates FMS; stress can actually block the healing of the central nervous system ravaged by FMS. To recover fully, you must learn to protect your energy and the vulnerable core of the condition: your central nervous system. This means unplugging from every possible source of unnecessary outside stress, be it a toxic job, marriage, friendship, or family member. The kinds of changes you need to make and whether they must be permanent or temporary depends on a number of factors: how seriously or chronically something or someone has been stressing you, how long you have been ill, how seriously ill you have become, and how long it will take your own body to heal.

After you have been unplugged from a dysfunctional relationship for a while and have made headway on your healing path, you will be able to tell whom you are strong enough to contact, how much contact is safe, and whom you really need to stay away from a while longer, maybe even permanently. You may grow and change, but others may not. Trust your instincts, honor your feelings, and do not allow guilt, false obligations, or misplaced responsibility to sabotage your health. Always do what is best for you.

You Deserve a Chance

You deserve every chance to regain your health and live your life in peace; you have every right to take charge of your life and choose to live it differently. Your ability to assess safety in your relationships will develop through the healing process. You will know when you are stronger whom you can have a connection with.

Emerging from this process with your health and a detached sense of loving compassion and forgiveness for others is a real possibility. Whether you choose to reconnect with a dysfunctional person, even in a very brief and detached way, is your decision. When you are healthy enough to reconnect with someone from your past, be careful not to fall into old patterns. By waiting until you are healthy and not allowing dysfunction to regain control, what was once an unhealthy relationship may turn into a wonderful one.

The last thing I want to say about leaving a dysfunctional relationship is this: you must create a strong support system and not tolerate any negativity or guilt trips from others about your decision. As long you understand what you need to do, you do not need to convince or persuade anyone. This is no one else's concern. It is important to find a supportive therapist to help you through this transition and a friend who is healthy enough psychologically to respect and support your decision without judging you; any form of nonjudgmental support will help.

Distancing yourself from stressful people, no matter who they are, may be necessary to get well. Even if you have to begin with all new friends or pick a new spiritual family, you will attract healthier people capable of respecting you and behaving appropriately. The bottom line is: if you really desire to heal, you must avoid those who drain your energy with the stress of abusive or destructive behavior.

After I detached from the dysfunctional relationships in my life, I grew to understand the importance of defining myself by my boundaries and surrounding myself with people who respect them. With my emotional needs met, I now felt free to concentrate on the physical part of my healing process.

Understanding the Dysfunction

Through therapy I have learned that in dysfunctional relationships there is very little expression of unselfish love. A therapist once told me that the dysfunctional home resembles a psychological war zone, and to grow up in this environment is like growing up on the front lines where you do not always know whom you can trust.

The chronic stress of this dysfunction can prevent the development and maintenance of a healthy balance between the mind, body, and spirit. The deprivation that occurs on all three levels can be devastating to a life. There is an old saying, "The only way out is through," and the only way through is by educating yourself, and, most importantly, applying what you learn to your life.

Learning to understand the dysfunction means you will be taking off blinders you may have unknowingly worn for a lifetime. Once you remove them you will no longer live partially in the dark. Seeing things illuminated for the first time means your eyes may need time to adjust before they can see clearly again, like walking out of a dimly lit room into full sunlight. But they will eventually adjust, you will eventually view things differently and, surprisingly, you will come to prefer it that way.

For me, I needed to learn to see each person in my life as they really are and understand what made them that way before I could understand myself. This process can be both surprising and painful; but this is a necessary step in determining which relationships cause the most undue stress. Your health is your responsibility, and as such, you must do everything possible to fight FMS and regain control of your life.

Though I often saw my dysfunctional relationships more clearly than others, I lacked sufficient understanding to relieve my anxiety about the feared gray areas and mysterious black holes. I could not fully see what was there until I stopped being blinded by my ignorance. In order to do this, I had to piece together my history. I needed certain mysteries to be solved. The story had to be told and it had to come to an end.

Getting Your History Straight

Getting your history straight is a very effective method for getting an accurate and balanced perspective of your life. Identifying the truth and seeing it laid down in black and white will set the past apart from your present and help you connect the dots of the mysterious, blurry picture called your life. Some mysteries may never be solved, but at least you will know this and can accept it. The rest can only be solved from your adult perspective and the life experience and understanding you lacked as a child.

Remembering your past through the limitations of a child's perspective will not help shed light on important events and can perpetuate unnecessary pain and illusion. Taking a look at your past through adult eyes will put things in their proper perspectives. Then you can see the past as a story that can be told, understood, and ended. While your story does not define who you are, the truth about your past will empower you to make wiser choices in the present, thus creating a better future. Begin this process by assembling as many pieces of the puzzle as you can.

Assembling the Puzzle Called Your Life

The easiest way to begin is by making a chronological list of the main events of your life. Be sure to include all physical injuries, especially those related to the neck and spine. Briefly list the memories, both positive and negative, that stand out the most from each year. Keep these memories as accurate as possible and try to leave out any embellishments, exaggerations, minimizations, assumptions, or spins made by yourself or others as the years have gone by. Focus on your own true experiences.

Remember, it is the truth that sets you free and brings you peace, not a facsimile. The truth here is going to be your best and most powerful friend. It does not matter if anyone else remembers things the way you do. Each person has his or her own reality, a collection of individual experiences and memories, which do not have to coincide with others. You can turn to others to check your facts and clarify hazy details, but to keep the integrity of your memories intact, do not share this list with anyone who may challenge the validity of what you have written.

Putting Together Your Health History

After you've completed listing your personal history, it is also helpful to put your health record in order. This may help you see a progressive pattern and give you an idea about when you began to exhibit fibromyalgia symptoms both physically and mentally. Keep it as simple and as accurate as possible with respect to your age and the health issues you had at that age. Physical manifestations of health issues have a pattern of their own. You will begin to recognize this pattern when you outline your health history.

Solving the Unsolved Mysteries

The last step in putting together the puzzle of your life is analyzing and reconciling the key unsolved mysteries linked to issues from your past and bringing them to their nearest and most logical conclusions. Pick the mysteries that seem to be linked with on-going themes of your life, such as psychological or emotional issues. Your themes may be different from others in your family, but if the experiences that brought about these themes were shared, then your themes may be similar.

Think back at the comments made by others about these issues and then think about what you actually remember. Apply the understanding of an adult to past events by looking at them with the common sense and perception you lacked as a child. This will bring light to many things which may have seemed unclear.

Question judgments made by others that you may have accepted as fact. Look back on your life with the attitude that anything was possible. Lay the events out in order and then decide what is most likely, knowing the people involved the way you do now. Patterns rarely change in people, especially in dysfunctional families, and behaviors can be predictable and consistent. It is always admirable to give the benefit of the doubt, but not when what is doubted has very little history of a benefit. Be consistent with reality and true to your recollections. Address the main issues most relevant to your life that seem to represent your own life-theme. These are the issues which will help you answer your most important questions.

Telling and Ending the Story

Before assembling a relevant story from these questions, first bear in mind the nature of the people involved and the credibility of their testimonies. Do not discount what someone has said simply because they may be dysfunctional; everyone, at some point, tells the truth. Your job is to decide who was telling it when these major life events occurred.

After doing this exercise, I was able to solve various mysteries and answer key questions pertaining to my life-themes. I came to realize that the lives of my parents and the choices they made long ago do not have to define me, nor do they determine my self-worth, and that I do not have to go through life being haunted by someone else's ghosts. As an adult, **I** am responsible for determining my self-worth, **my** truth determines who I am, and what I choose to do or not do is my responsibility.

After two years of therapy, guided education, and forty plus books on human psychology, I can now see my parents with the compassion, understanding, and forgiveness of an adult, rather than with the grief of a child. Not everyone realizes that life is a series of choices, and that even though we cannot always control what happens, how we choose to respond is within our control and is our responsibility.

We are all either limited or freed by our awareness of the power of choice, and sadly so many people through ignorance are prisoners of themselves, as I once was. The only way out of this prison is to choose to expand your understanding, apply what you learn to your life, and make wiser choices. Now that I understand it, I truly believe the best choice I can make is to say goodbye to the past. I take what I have learned as a gift and move forward in life with a clear and peaceful mind, a calm central nervous system, a warm, whole heart, and greater knowledge of myself and others. The wisdom I have gained from viewing the past as an informed adult will guide me through the rest of my life.

I realize there are a lot of jokes about being in therapy and blaming your parents, but therapy is not about blame. It is about understanding yourself, the past, and the people in it so you can take responsibility for your life and learn to take better care of yourself and the people you love. This kind of control only comes from healing the wounds of the past through the emotional and intellectual adventures of psychotherapy and guided education.

Now I rarely visit the past, except to reference it to make decisions in the present. When I think of my family, the compassion I feel for all of us spreads over my life like a healing salve and is merged into my generalized compassion for all the suffering souls on the planet.

I am securely on the path of maintaining my health and recovery, and I no longer allow anything to drain my life force energy or disrupt my serenity and happiness in the present. The past can be like a giant suction hose attached to a powerful vacuum cleaner; when you maintain a close connection with it, it can suck your life force energy right down its long unyielding tube into the bottom of a dark bag full of debris and bacteria where nothing from the present can live. Detaching from this hose will return to you a vital life force you did not even know you were missing, a force that you must have if you are going to get well from FMS. It is a fact that the farther away I get from my past, the more energy I have for healing in the present.

I heard Dr. Carolyn Myss, PhD, who is a known medical intuit and healer, say in one of her PBS-TV lectures, "If you want to heal, you must chart a course far away from the past and into the future." In order to do this, the past must no longer be your reality; you must live in the present. Living in the present entails not only being in the moment, but appreciating it as well. An attitude of appreciation is being grateful for the many blessings in your life as well as respecting life's many mysteries. This respect means having a healthy understanding that not all mysteries can be solved; some are simply there for us to observe and to be a part of for a time, and only exist for us to learn to live within life's mysteries as gracefully as possible. The past no longer has any living reality for me. Only the present is real, and in the present I am very blessed. My many blessings are my husband, his kids, my pets and my loving friends, and family members I have been able to reconnect with in healthy loving detachment.

Life can really be as simple as that. From what I have experienced and learned so far, I now look out the windows of my here and now and I marvel at how wonderful life can be when you make the right choices. In his book, *The Power of Now*, the wonderful modern-day spiritual leader and teacher Eckhart Tolle says, "The only sane way to live is in complete acceptance of what is – and know that it is neither good nor bad, but a part of a higher good, the higher good that has no opposite. The conflict within you ceases when the demands and expectations of your mind no longer clash with what is. Accept what is. Do what you have to do, but accept what is."

So go on and do what you have to do to heal yourself, and accept everything else as a part of the higher good. Start by educating yourself in all that you need to understand so you can cure this illness thoroughly. This book is the story of my journey and how I arrived back to this wonderful place called health. I hope with all my heart my story inspires others to step onto their own healing paths, take charge of their lives and their conditions, and discover the courage within them to make the choices that work to cure chronic FMS.

Comes the Dawn

After a while you learn the subtle difference
Between holding a hand and chaining a soul,
And you learn that love doesn't mean leaning
And company doesn't mean security,
And you begin to learn that kisses aren't contracts
And presents aren't promises,
And you begin to accept your defeats
With your head up and your eyes open
With the grace of a woman, not the grief of a child,
And you learn to build all your roads on today
Because tomorrow's ground is too uncertain for plans.
And futures have a way of falling down in mid-flight.
After a while you learn
That even sunshine burns if you get too much.
So you plant your own garden and decorate your own soul,
Instead of waiting for someone to bring you flowers.
And you learn that you really can endure …….
That you really are strong,
And you really do have worth.
And you learn and learn …….
With every goodbye, you learn.

--Virginia Shopstall

Chapter Two
Boundaries

Gaining Control Over Your Life

Someone with chronic FMS must employ healthy, functional internal and external boundaries in order to gain control over their life and reduce stress. People who are brought up in a dysfunctional family often enter into adulthood with little or no knowledge of the existence of boundaries and also lack an understanding of the importance of functional boundaries as an essential component in their relationships with others. Lack of boundaries is central to dysfunctional behavior and can seriously prevent a person from maturing into a functional, healthy adult. People who have grown up without boundaries often lose their sense of self in the resulting trauma, are often unable to recognize the presence or absence of abuse, and do not possess the ability to gain control over their lives.

Therefore, establishing healthy boundaries is imperative for self-protection and the development of a mature, healthy sense of self. Self-awareness, self-control, memory, and reasoning are higher mental functions. Mental maturity includes establishing healthy boundaries and the self-awareness that comes as a result of having them, and can be measured by the increase of these functions, just as mental degradation can be measured by their absence or loss.

There is a saying in Buddhism, "To say no means you have to know what yes is." It is within the process of figuring out what you do not want that you figure out what you do want. Having functional boundaries means saying no to what you don't want as easily as saying yes to what you want. Functional boundaries are also imperative to psychological, spiritual, and physical healing because they protect against the forces of destructive behavior that is often a bi-product of mental illness. The most effective way to protect your self against someone who is behaving badly and causing you undue stress is to utilize a system of personal boundaries that combines internal and external limits. Establishing a "code of honor" for yourself in the form of a system of boundaries will move you toward self-discovery and spiritual maturity. In this age of consciousness, the ideas that come to us from quantum physics, Zen Buddhism, psychology, etc., are meant to be applied to our lives in ways that propel us forward into our natural evolution as a species. These ideas are meant to guide us and change us. Boundaries are the most basic foundation for this process of personal discovery, change, enlightenment, and evolution.

Adults have boundaries and they respect the boundaries of others, even when they do not understand the whys and wherefores. Healthy adults do not expect others to sacrifice themselves to their selfish demands or needs, and appreciate and respect the rights and freedoms of others to live their lives as they see fit. When you develop healthy boundaries and join the ranks of boundary lovers, these are the people who you want to surround yourself with because they will respect and support your quest for emotional and physical health and can cheerfully say to your no thank you, "Okay, we'll miss seeing you this time but we'll catch you another time."

When you come across people who become angry or hostile when you say "no" or "no thank you," set appropriate boundaries against them and let them go their own way. You are not responsible to engage in an argument or discussion to make someone who is being intrusive understand your private business, or convince them of your reasons for setting a personal limit. Adults keep their own counsel and are not accountable to anyone else for their personal decisions regarding their wellbeing and safety. You do not have to explain yourself to anyone; however, if you wish to explain your reasons to someone whom you are safe or intimate with who respects you, for the sake of sharing, do so. While it is not a requirement to explain your boundaries, the act of confiding in a trusted friend or loved one always helps make the boundary-making process a bit easier.

Boundaries

Boundaries are like a fence around your property; they protect everything that you value and prevent others from trespassing on your rights and freedoms. When your fence has gaping holes of ambiguity, any intrusive element can enter undetected. This is why it's so important to know your boundaries before they are confronted. In addition to strong protection, your fence can have a locked gate leading in and out of your life and personal space. You not only have the right to decide where and how far out to put your fences, you can also decide when to unlock the gate and let someone in.

These decisions are yours to make. There will always be outside pressure to set your boundaries in ways that benefit others, but if you use your good judgment and follow through with your right to make and maintain boundaries, you can keep yourself at a safe distance from all that will harm your recovery.

Remember one thing: in addition to keeping unwanted elements out, your boundaries keep you in. Sometimes this is necessary; however, living your whole life behind a fence with a locked gate can be very lonely. What I am talking about here is risk. There are times to close the gate and lock it and there are times to unlock it and let people and events into your life. There are no guarantees that you will not get hurt when you do this, but in order to grow you must be open to new experiences. The key here is to know when the risk is worth it. Not every person or situation requires a locked gate. Over time, you will learn to discern when and with whom a locked gate is necessary. When it is, you must endure the difficulties of standing by your decision and not cave in to the gears, scorns, and guilt trips that are bound to come your way. Staying resolute is key to your recovery. You are the keeper of your mind, your body, and your soul. You are responsible for your life and the choices you make. This is an inescapable part of having been given the gift of life. Making these choices, however uncertain they may seem at times, is always worth the effort!

Definition and Purpose of Boundaries

Boundaries are a system of internal and external limits that enables a person to gain some control over the effect they have on others and others have on them. The specific purpose of a boundary is to provide a framework that provides a clear sense of your reality and a clear sense of yourself. There are four areas of boundaries that define and contain your reality and who you are apart from others.

Boundaries Deal With Four Areas

- Limits you set for your physical body (how you appear).
- Your thoughts (how you interpret what you experience and the meaning you assign it).
- Your feelings (emotions resulting from thoughts and/or information collected by your body - "body intelligence").
- Your behavior (what you choose to do or not do).

Your reality consists of how you look, how you feel, how you think, and what you do or do not do. This self-defined reality is different for each person. Some people have a clear and healthy system of boundaries in place while others, such as those who suffer from codependency, lack a functional system of boundaries and, as a result, do not have an accurate view of themselves or their reality.

Moreover, these people have their internal boundary in reverse, which tells them they are responsible for the feelings and choices of others and that others are responsible for theirs. This reversal results in the misplacement of responsibility, causing people to stress over things they cannot control and to feel victimized by the actions of others. The victim role is when a person is being their most immature and dysfunctional.

When our internal and external boundaries are functioning strongly and simultaneously, the spiritual boundary is automatically present and is very powerful. Then when we share our lives with others we can feel spiritually connected to all who share the same respect for our personal boundaries as we do for theirs. This ability is what God intends for us; the ability to understand that we are all connected through the same life force energy, yet are simultaneously divided by our physical bodies and responsibility for self-care.

Understanding External and Internal Boundaries

External: External boundaries have to do with protecting the body by keeping it healthy and safe from harm. This applies to both non-sexual and sexual situations and deals with decisions, such as when and how close you get to another person physically and when and who gets to touch you. These boundaries are meant to control distance and touch.

Internal: Internal boundaries have to do with owning your responsibility for your choices in thought and action even when your are responding to someone else. Although we need to be sensitive to the effect we have on others if we want to be in relationships, the only time we are responsible for the feelings of another is when we are disrespectful, abusive, or harmful. Then we must take responsibility, show remorse, and make amends.

We cannot always change the way others assign meaning to what we say or do, or how they choose to feel about us. There is an old saying, "What other people think of you is none of your business!" All we can do is make sure we are not an offender and try to do no harm. Whenever a person has committed a major offense, they are accountable for it. They are then obliged to make amends, which means taking personal responsibility for their behavior, showing remorse, and promising to work hard at never doing it again. If they are not willing to do this then they are not capable of a healthy adult relationship. It then becomes necessary to evaluate and assess the psychological health and safety of those you are attempting to have a relationship with and the nature of the relationship you can have with them, if any.

Evaluating External Boundaries

- The healthy, intact external boundary constantly evaluates distance and touch in your interactions with others. You protect yourself by controlling how far away you are from someone and whether or not you allow them to touch you. You are still somewhat vulnerable to the actions of others.
- The non-existent external boundary is when you do not evaluate distance or touch in your interaction with others and have no awareness that something is lacking. You are completely vulnerable, as you do not have a boundary to protect you from the actions of others.
- The intermittent boundary only provides you with partial protection, as it sometimes involves a healthy boundary and sometimes involves either a partial boundary or no boundary at all. This may happen for several reasons: you may not yet understand how to maintain your boundaries no matter who you are with, fatigue may weaken your resolve, or sickness may drain you of the energy required to constantly keep your boundaries intact.
- The extreme alternating external boundary is continually alternating between having no boundaries at all to utilizing walls. This is dangerous because you go from allowing everyone in to allowing no one in. Not only does this affect your well-being, it can drive off people who could be positive influences in your life.
- Finally, the perpetual wall. Walls provide complete protection, allowing no intimacy, and should always be used when you are interacting with chronic or extreme offenders. Walls consist of extremes in behavior that completely separate you from others such as anger, humor, talking, silence, politeness or distance. These behaviors in extreme allow no intimate contact and you are completely protected, contained, and isolated; however, they take an enormous amount of energy to maintain. The least draining is physical distance.

Evaluating Internal Boundaries

- The healthy, intact internal boundary is functioning when you are taking responsibility for yourself and your reality and allowing others to be responsible for theirs. At the same time, you are able to be sensitive to the effects you have on others and can freely and moderately communicate the effects that others have on you.

- Remember, adults keep their own council and take action for self-care.
- The non-existent internal boundary is when the boundary of responsibility is reversed, where you blame others for your reality and you blame yourself for theirs. This is the proverbial blame game that is played by every victim and gets to be a real drag.
- The intermittent internal boundary functions inconsistently, depending on internal and external circumstances: how you feel, where you are and whom you are with. Ideally, this boundary should be functioning as consistently as possible.
- Finally, there is the internal wall. The internal wall occurs when you completely shut yourself in and everyone else out; you do not open up to anyone and you show no interest in others.

Intermittent boundaries indicate holes in your metaphorical fences. Pay attention to what happens to your boundaries when you are around certain people or in certain situations that seem to cause them to function intermittently. Learning to utilize consistent boundaries is like learning to play a musical instrument; all it takes is practice, practice, practice and will soon come naturally. The holes in your fences will eventually be repaired and you will be protected most of the time.

No one has boundaries that are fully functional all of the time. Learning to be responsible for your own reality is the key to being an adult and is an important goal to set for yourself. Nobody can be human, endure stress and illness and the ups and downs of life, and keep a perfect boundary system going all the time. Just practice doing your best and you will become more aware in time. Remember, practicing boundaries at times in a situation that requires them will make your boundary setting skills stronger than if you never practice using them at all.

Healthy Models for Appropriate Boundary Setting

The Bible is the most popular book ever written and, with the right interpretation, can provide healthy role models for appropriate boundary setting. Matthew 18: 15-18 says, "Moreover if thy brother shall trespass against thee, go and tell him his fault between thee and him alone; if he shall hear thee, thou hast gained thy brother. But if he will not hear thee, then take with thee one or two more that in the mouth of two or three witnesses, every word may be established. And if he shall neglect to hear them, tell it unto the church: but if he neglects to hear the church, let him be unto thee as a heathen man and a publican. Verily I say unto you, whatsoever ye shall bind on earth shall be bound in heaven: and whatsoever ye shall loose on earth shall be loosed in heaven." This means some people will get to be in your life while others will not. It is just the way a healthy adult world works, so set boundaries and see who gets to stay.

All adults are responsible for both setting and honoring boundaries. In setting boundaries, you neither owe an explanation nor do you require permission to set them. Boundaries are for self-preservation and they do not have to be explained.

Honoring boundaries, whether they are your own internal boundaries or the external boundaries of others, is something adults do. Honoring the boundaries of others should not be seen as a "favor" given with guilt messages or false debt attached.

Boundaries are to be celebrated in ourselves and in others as good self-care. Healthy adults who take good care of themselves love the boundaries of others. They respect and honor them without complaint and make an honest and willing effort to remember them.

If you are faced with a chronic boundary violator, you can remind them a couple of times and if they continue to violate your boundaries or make no effort to remember it, then it is appropriate to distance yourself from them. Chronic boundary violators are not capable of healthy intimate relationships.

Give your relationships the litmus test of boundaries and carefully observe how they are honored. If your boundaries are ignored, resented, or honored with complaints about how inconvenient or disagreeable they are, then the quality of your relationship with that person is not healthy. Find out with whom you can have a healthy adult relationship and whom you cannot. There are plenty of healthy boundary lovers out there who can honor and celebrate your boundaries without judging you and can set boundaries for themselves graciously and respectfully and make an effort to remember yours. Naturally, children do not have the capacity to always remember boundaries. Patience and consequences are therefore required to help them learn the importance of honoring boundaries so they can become adults who are capable of loving, intimate relationships. Remember that boundaries exist to teach "self-control" and not "other-control."

Also, remember you do not owe anyone an explanation for setting a boundary. You may choose to offer an explanation if you feel they are capable of understanding it and wish to maintain some closeness with that person; however, if you suspect a person is not capable of understanding your reasons, or from past experience has shown that they are not, you may choose to offer no explanation whatsoever.

An immature person would rather have you accommodate or enable their inappropriate behaviors and selfish demands than have you take the healthier position of setting up boundaries against them.   The book *Boundaries,* by Cloud and Townsend, states, "I would rather be around people who are capable of taking personal responsibility and who honestly fail me, and can own their behavior (admit to it), apologize, make amends (promise to try in earnest never to do it again) and repent (make a true change in direction) than people who dishonestly deny ever having hurt me and have no intension of taking personal responsibility for their behavior or doing better in the future." I whole-heartedly agree!

How to Set Boundaries

The word "no" is the most effective and most solid of boundaries. There are not any ifs, ands, or buts about it and it is very clear and non-negotiable. Sometimes, based on the information at hand, a "no" boundary is required. When it is, you must do your part and stand by your boundary. This is not to say when you receive new information you may not decide to change your mind and adjust your boundary to some degree. You most certainly may. The point here is that **you** are in control of your boundary and can change it according to your on-going assessment. However, if no new information comes to you warranting a practical change or adjustment, then your boundary should be upheld.

Upholding your boundary is the beginning of the work of boundary setting. This means resisting the demands and guilt trips laid on you by others, resisting giving up your moral principals out of fear of rejection, condemnation, or loneliness, and resisting the temptation to abandon your position out of fatigue.

You must base all of your decisions in life, including your reasons for setting a boundary, on what you truly think, feel, and believe. Otherwise, you will be abandoning yourself time and again in the most fundamental way possible. You will be abandoning your responsibility for self-preservation, which can be seriously self-destructive.

People who are passive-compliant are not able to say no. They believe that they either belong to others or do not have the right to say no. As a result, they are chronically dishonest both with themselves and with others.   There is an old joke about the passive-compliant: Question: "What happens when a passive-compliant meets an egocentric-controller?" Answer: "They get married." The tragic reality is that the passive-compliant usually does not realize they are in an abusive or destructive relationship until it is too late, if ever.

We all share the same responsibility to grow up into mature adults and set boundaries to preserve our healthy lives. We must learn to value the importance of distancing ourselves from or letting go of people who cannot or will not love and respect our "no." People who attempt to manipulate you out of your "no" often become angry and act as if something is being done "to them" when in reality something is not being done "for them."

Mature adults with good boundaries use the word "no" as easily and as automatically as they use the word "yes" without any guilt, animosity, or second thoughts. They are as gracious and accepting of the boundaries of others as they are in the way they set boundaries for themselves. It is important to understand that boundaries protect love, create intimacy, allow responsibility to lie with the correct people, and force people to be mature and develop self-control instead of trying to control others. Without boundaries, relationships cannot work and no one can be at ease, happy, or healthy.

Setting boundaries can be as easy as politely saying, "Thank you, but I'm not up to it just now. Maybe some other time," or "I'd rather not, thank you." If someone does not respect the boundaries you have in place you can be a little more aggressive in your refusal, but do not waste your energy trying to appease them. Set your boundary and walk away from the situation; do not cause yourself any undue stress by trying to justify yourself to someone else. On the other hand, boundaries can be enjoyable between healthy adults, and can even make you closer through your mutual respect for their importance. I once knew a lady who could set boundaries so easily and graciously you did not even know she had done it.

A strong system of healthy external and internal boundaries is the only way we can keep ourselves safe from harm and become mature, happy, functioning adults who are capable of loving, intimate relationships. Boundaries protect us from people who are rude, intrusive, manipulative, deceitful, and judgmental. They protect us from those who use lies, guilt, coercion, and emotional blackmail to control and use others to meet their selfish needs. Learn to recognize these destructive behaviors and to say no to them.

Exercise your God-given right to self-preservation and self-actualization. Set a healthy example for your kids by providing them with an example of how to set and maintain boundaries. By doing so, you will be prepared to face whatever challenge comes your way without compromising your healing process. Become a liver of the way of boundaries and give your adult relationships the litmus test of boundaries. You will attract like-minded people who can contribute to your life in a positive way. Get with it! Get boundaries! And be aware of what to expect.

What to Expect

When you enforce your boundaries for the first time, people are going to react in a variety of ways. Mature, healthy adults will respect your decisions, but some people will not be so supportive. People who have grown up in dysfunction have emotional and psychological needs that others do not, and if separation from you will mean that their needs will not be met, they will not be happy to see you distance yourself. If they try to send you a guilt trip, don't pack your bags. Hold tight and maintain your position.

When you apply healthy standards to unhealthy people it is going to cause pain and anger, like fitting them with new shoes that need braking in. If you are not strong in your decision to lead a healthy life, this situation could escalate and cause an immense amount of negativity and stress. Just remember: there is no arguing. You do not owe anyone an explanation, and should not allow them to force you to give one. People are going to think what they need to for their own reasons, so let them. Allow them their discomfort, maintain your boundaries and healthier values anyway.

There is another, deeper reason for the inevitable resistance and unpleasantness you are sure to encounter. When someone educates themself and attempts to apply what they learn, it can threaten the unconscious psychological core of someone else who behaves inappropriately. When someone changes and stops participating in dysfunctional behavior, it alters the entire dynamic of the relationship.

A dysfunctional family is like a rusty, rigid mobile. An "immobile mobile," so to speak. When one piece of the mobile oils up, breaks loose, and changes position, the other pieces of the mobile become strained and creaky and are forced into changing positions relative to each other, in an attempt to maintain some kind of balance. They crack and they squeak and they jerk about in unwieldy ways. This causes a ripple effect of discomfort and anger because this change was imposed upon them and not made by choice.

When someone can predict how you will act or react, they feel they have some control over you. When you begin to set boundaries and limits to protect yourself and stop participating in unhealthy behavior, you are no longer predictable to them, and therefore no longer easy for them to manipulate or control. By honestly defining yourself by your boundaries when before you had none, they feel you have changed and not in a good way. The negative reactions of others are a positive sign that you are on the right track.

When you have maintained a healthier lifestyle long enough, former relationship dynamics will change. If you are not outright rejected, you may become a source of irritation and discomfort. Do not be discouraged. Sooner or later, those who are capable of a healthy relationship will understand what you are doing and respect you for it.

The ones who truly love you will come around and tolerate your boundaries, even if they don't understand them. Others will maintain their anger, which stems from a misunderstanding of what you are trying to do. While you see your actions as positive ways to support your health, they may see your actions as a personal commentary on their character. This may cause them to think badly of you, but hopefully, with time, they can learn to understand what you are doing. Remember the old saying, "What other people think of you is none of your business, nor is it your problem." Depending on how enmeshed or central a player you have been in a dysfunctional relationship, your pulling out of the game quietly and solidly may or may not have an effect on the way others relate. This is none of your business. Concentrate on yourself.

It is important to understand that all this "re-activeness" toward your sudden honesty and boundary setting is going to be natural and, more importantly, unconscious. You will be threatening the way in which others view their lives, their relationships, and their reality. This can be terrifying to them, and in truth can constitute a very real threat of unconscious psychological annihilation. This death of self naturally precedes the birth of a new and healthier self, but this does not make the process any less terrifying. Consider verbal attacks as merely animal instincts; when an animal, any animal, feels cornered it will naturally and automatically attack as a primal survival response. So naturally those you set boundaries against are going to resist you, and the most immature and unconscious ones will feel their only option is to attack. These are the major offenders.

Try to have compassion and patience, and allow others to formulate their own opinions about how your actions affect them. They have a right to react to your actions in their own ways, and you have a right to not allow these reactions to get in the way of your healing process, and never tolerate abuse. Depending on how severely people react, you may need to distance yourself from them for a while, a few years, or even permanently. Maintain your boundaries, wait and see what happens, and let the chips fall where they may! Bruce Barton once said, "Nothing splendid has ever been achieved except by those who dared believe that something inside them was superior to circumstance." Rise above it, be true to yourself, and stick to your boundaries.

Do not be surprised when your boundaries are tested, violated, or only intermittently honored. This is natural. When people react badly to you, pay attention to what it is you are doing that causes them to react in this way. Both sides are responsible to watch how they behave and to not antagonize others.

You cannot expect other people to behave appropriately and honor your boundaries if you are not willing to do the same. When you make an agreement with someone about a limit you need, you must try to stay within that limit yourself. Anatole France said, "To accomplish great things we must not only act, but dream. Not only plan, but also believe." We must act as though we believe that the dream of a better, healthier self can emerge from what we are now and that there is a way to achieve this goal. Dream of a better life, educate yourself about what is healthy and what is not, take action by applying what you learn, and things will only get better.

When you suddenly become a boundary setter you become like a gazelle in a lion's den, and it can be difficult to protect yourself. Zoos keep the gazelles and lions separated for good reason. The first boundaries you set will simply serve as a way to determine who can and cannot respect them without hostility or abuse. This is the only way to find out with whom you can be in contact and with whom you need to distance yourself for the sake of your own health. This is the most important step on the path to curing FMS because eliminating unnecessary stress is crucial to healing the central nervous system. You cannot get well without doing this first and almost nothing is more stressful and exhausting than participating in dysfunctional relationships.

The more stress you are able to take out of your life the better your healing process will progress. There are many different kinds of negative behaviors associated with dysfunction, and you should become familiar with when and how they occur. Anticipating these behaviors will help you to avoid unnecessary confrontations. A good therapist can help you work through your relationships and teach you how to distance yourself in a healthy, stress reducing way. When you are met with a negative reaction to your boundaries, understand that a person who reacts in such a way may feel threatened. You are causing them to look at something they may not want to see, but their unwillingness to face your reality is not something that you can control. Again, allow them their discomfort and distance yourself; respect their right to be who they are.

There is a chance that a gracious and appropriate boundary will be accepted and respected with no hassles. However, if a boundary is met with hostility or anger, then once again, distance yourself. Remember that unless it will promote understanding, you do not need to explain your reasons for setting a boundary; explaining boundaries to people who have no respect for your right to set them is a misuse of energy and will cause unnecessary stress. You cannot afford to waste this energy during the healing process.

There will be times when people do not understand why you are setting boundaries, or do not understand that these boundaries apply to them. In either case, these people may be hurt and respond to your actions in negative ways. Do not be discouraged by the negativity. If you know these boundaries are necessary for your recovery, do not back down. All you can do is take responsibility for your own behavior; you cannot be held responsible for the way others feel about your actions. By explaining yourself you may simply cause more of an argument, so do not try and justify anything unless the other person is understanding enough to benefit from it. Only use your energy when it will be useful, and do not give in to senseless arguments.

While others should respect the boundaries you set, you should set them in a respectful way. Stating a blameless, non-judgmental boundary can be as simple as saying, "No, I don't feel good about this," or "No, this just doesn't feel right to me," or "It's best for me if I stop right here," or "I don't feel I can do this anymore," or "Excuse me but I need to get some space for a while," or "Let's not talk about the past. Let's stick to the present," or "I'm sorry you feel that way, but it doesn't change things for me." Do not be spiteful or pass blame when you set your boundaries, instead be honest and polite. Hold your position and be responsible for the way you set boundaries and for how you uphold them.

I Say Goodbye

I say goodbye to an innocent buried
I say goodbye to a childhood missed
I say goodbye to the unseen blossom
To the twisted vine by the dew not kissed
I say goodbye to a poisoned youth
I say goodbye as it finally ends
I turn my back and am not defeated
I boldly go where the road now bends
I say goodbye to the beguiled young beauty
I say goodbye as she lived unknown
I say goodbye to old dreams escaping
To the pearl whose host was blindly sewn
I say goodbye to the misplaced promise
I say goodbye to the years that died
To the terror, and mercy, and pain repeated
To the untrained pilot who charmed and lied
I say goodbye to the spirit shredder
To the Grizzly's claw as its grasp uncurls
I see its retreat and its dissipation
And the lifeless pose of its face unfurled
I say goodbye to the unknown God
To the un-kept faith and the un-felt trust
To the blind man's staff, to the warlord's treasure
I leap from the mountain, as I know I must.

Valerie Lumley

Chapter Three
Authentic Forgiveness

A physical necessity meant to cleanse, not absolve

One of the most important components of inner peace is authentic forgiveness. Forgiving your transgressors relieves your soul of the burden of wounded debt. It clears the mind, the body, and the spirit of the weight of the past, and allows you to achieve inner peace. This is what an FMS sufferer needs most: the peace of being psychologically and emotionally free so that their body can focus its energy on the healing process. FMS lives inside the central nervous system, causing it to become hyperactive and hypersensitive. The body needs every ounce of energy to fight off the system-wide ravages of this disease.

Authentic forgiveness is a process, not an event, and is also a widely misunderstood pathway. There is so much confusion about forgiveness, about who deserves it and how one goes about giving it, and why. When someone takes personal responsibility for their behavior, apologizes sincerely, and promises to do better, forgiving them can be a relatively easy process.

Conversely, an insincere apology or the absence of from a person who has no intention of taking responsibility by owning up to their actions and behavior can make things much worse. In this case, the person who committed the offense does not care whether or not you forgive them, and forgiveness now becomes a function for your own peace of mind. The act of forgiveness is ultimately meant to cleanse the heart of the person doing the forgiving rather than absolving the forgiven transgressor of their personal responsibility. I want to sort all this out and clear a pathway to forgiveness to help make it seem accessible, understandable and practical.

In all of our relationships, both healthy and dysfunctional, we always hurt the one we love. Forgiveness is a necessary requirement for a healthy mind, body, and spirit. You can use forgiveness as a tool to begin healing the wounds inflicted in your past; forgiving someone who hurt you will free you from harbored anger and will help you learn to set up healthy, protective boundaries.

Another tool like forgiveness is understanding. You can use acquired understanding to find peace with your past and learn to live better in the present and future. When you understand the people and events in the past, you will be able to focus your energy on your healing process rather than emotional turmoil; therefore, the process of authentically forgiving your transgressors through understanding becomes a physical necessity. Actor Mickey Rooney said, "Forgiveness is the only real power we have." I would like to add that we also have the power to direct our lives by our choices, and authentic forgiveness is a choice like everything else.

Keep in mind that the process of forgiving is not always fast or easy. The time and effort it takes to authentically forgive someone varies based on the size of the transgression, the severity of the wound, and the amount of time that the harm has lasted. I feel the deeper wounds, especially those repeatedly inflicted over a long period of time, can take the longest to forgive. However long it takes to arrive at authentic forgiveness, be it a few minutes, hours, years, or even a lifetime, the process is essentially the same. The process of authentic forgiveness is accomplished in the following ways and begins with detachment on all levels.

Detachment on All Levels

1) Physical Detachment

In the case of severe or chronic abuse, it may be necessary to create a physical boundary of space and time. This boundary should precede all others. It should initially preclude contact of any kind with the offender, including physical contact, phone calls, letters, and messages, even those sent through others. Only discuss this individual or individuals with those inside your immediate support group, such as your therapist, spouse, or a close friend.

It is wise to utilize the support of a good therapist. Life changing decisions need guidance, and a good therapist can help prevent you from abandoning yourself through this process out of fear, guilt, false-obligation, outside attacks, or separation anxiety. The physical boundary does not always need to be permanent, although in some cases it does.

2) Psychological Detachment

It is necessary to educate yourself thoroughly and become an expert on the nature of your injuries, the effects your injuries have had on your life, and the origin and cause of the injuries you have suffered. A good therapist can guide you through this process and recommend resources, such as books, that will help with your specific situation. Randomly reading from the self-help section of your local bookstore can become confusing, disturbing, and very time consuming. The right books at the right time will give the necessary understanding and added strength and support.

While you are learning to understand the nature of your injuries you will simultaneously be learning to understand yourself. To "know thy self" is a very powerful way to be clear and certain about your reality. A lot of peace and security comes from knowing yourself and being clear in how you feel about things. This peace can open you up to the right choices and allow you to put things into their natural perspective.

Learning to recognize and understand the effects your injuries have had on your life can make sense of how you feel about things today, and learning new terms will enable you to discuss it clearly. This can help you recognize and identify your feelings in the present and separate them from things that closely resemble the past.

If the present reminds you of the past in some way, you can choose to respond more appropriately by applying what you have learned from your past experiences. Separating the present from the past allows you to keep current events in their proper perspective so you can respond appropriately and proportionately.

Finally, understanding the cause and origin of your injuries includes learning to understand the true nature and personal dynamics of the people who have harmed you. This will be very helpful in separating yourself from them psychologically, as it will help you see yourself and them objectively as individuals, enable you to draw a line between where you end and where they begin, and will give you the strong sense of separateness you will need to successfully detach.

3) Spiritual Detachment

It is extremely helpful to acknowledge the fact that arriving at authentic forgiveness by detaching physically, psychologically, and spiritually is healing to the body, mind, and the evolving soul. This evolution is most commonly referred to as the "spiritual growth process," and is meant to continue naturally throughout life. Recognizing the evolutionary nature of your soul and the higher power that created it is a very important step.

Believing that one spirit cannot release itself from another is incorrect conditioning. We are all keepers of our own souls with the power to release ourselves from the grip of pain inflicted on us by others. One way to do this is symbolically laying them onto the Alter and giving them to God with as much love and forgiveness as possible. God is ultimately responsible for guiding and forgiving them. When you are not yet ready to forgive, God will always be. We should focus our energy on the process of personal growth and healing.

Forgiveness is part of this process. By forgiving someone, you remove the burden of their transgression from your shoulders, an action which brings forth a peaceful form of detachment and allows you to focus your strength on beating FMS. Forgiveness also puts responsibility in the appropriate places by making the transgressor responsible for their soul and you responsible for yours.

Take Time

Allow time for your new detachment to take hold and settle in; time to absorb and process all that you are learning so that it becomes an integral part of yourself and your life; time to learn to live life differently and get used to the strange peace that accompanies detachment. If you have had to distance yourself from someone, take time to fill this new space with healthier people and occupations; time to discover the wounded self now healing, now being redefined, now expanding and creating a new healthier identity; time to create a new relationship with God; time to experience your life within the limitless bounds of freedom that comes with detachment; time to experience the newfound energy that was once chronically depleted by tolerating the pain of inappropriate attachments.

Emotional, physical, and spiritual pain can deplete your energy at an enormous cost to your biological balance. Furthermore, it can alter who you are and gradually collapse you into resignation, complacency, and stagnation. It can rob you of your joy and ability to develop your unique gifts and full potential. Chronic emotional pain can so consume you that your life can seem to be merely passing by. This is the saga of the unfulfilled life and the unevolved spirit. Do not allow this to happen to you. Take the time you need to walk away from relationship dysfunction and build yourself a healthier life.

Honor Thyself

Honoring yourself means to acknowledge, validate, and experience your feelings exactly as they are. Experience them in all their complexity or simplicity and allow them to surface uncensored. What you feel may be painful, frightening and confusing, but this is normal. Pay attention to this confusion, as it is important to work out things that bother you. Your connection with yourself is experience through these feelings, so sorting them out is very important. In any way you can, feel your emotions, suffer through them, tolerate the discomfort they cause, allow them all to well up and wash them away with tears if necessary. Process them out of you instead of holding them in. The combined physical, emotional, and psychological pain of FMS is like no other. Release it.

Painful feelings have a life of their own. They may take a while to release, sort out, identify, and express, but be assured. Painful feelings cannot sustain themselves unless you hold them back or choose not to acknowledge and express them when appropriate. When you let painful feelings surface and make themselves known they will naturally dissipate. Conversely, when you hold them back, they grow in intensity and can eventually permeate your entire body. Pent up emotional pain tends to warp, mutate, and combine with other feelings, eventually becoming unrecognizable and developing the power to chain your mind and oppress your soul.

Ignoring and/or suppressing your feelings ultimately blocks grace, joy, and serendipity (the unsolicited gifts of life). Dishonoring your feelings in this way can rob you of everything worthwhile that life has to offer. The cost of holding your feelings back and blocking their expression is said to be a thousand times greater than the pain and stress that comes from honoring and experiencing them in a healthy way.

It is said there is nothing more painful than unexpressed feelings. Experiencing their expression and all they have to teach, and releasing them to make room for a new and expanding self, will enable you to come out on the other side of this process with more compassion for yourself and for the suffering of others. You have everything to gain from honoring your feelings and everything to loose by not.

"You are a child of the universe, no less than the trees and the stars; you have the right to be here" – Desiderata. You have the right to be who you are, feel what you feel, think what you think, and live your own life as you choose as a growing, flourishing, ever expanding human being with a peaceful mind, a joyful heart, and fulfilled soul.

"The only way out is through." Go into and through your feelings. There is no right or wrong way to feel. Every feeling has a reason. It may be terrifying or overwhelming at times, but you can come out safely on the other side. You can come out of the darkness and into the light with the peace of knowing what is deep within you, hiding nothing, seeing clearly, being honest with yourself and others, and living your life as a gift that has been given to you.

Assessing Your Reality

You must make a realistic assessment of your life. Detachment is a tool that allows you to stand back far enough to take a good look at the big picture and see all of it at once, probably for the first time. Suppressed, unprocessed emotional pain can create tunnel vision and put narrow blinders over your view of life. When someone or something is harming you, your energy becomes significantly depleted by the task of surviving, leaving little or no energy for assessing the very circumstances you are trying to survive.

Survival is naturally our number one priority, and when we are stuck in survival mode our assessment skills can become overshadowed, blurring our vision of reality. Under these conditions, making a realistic assessment of the harsh realities of your suffering can be extremely difficult. Do not let your vision be skewed by pain. Try and see through it to determine how to best identify and overcome your discomfort.

When someone presents a threat to your health, be it psychological, physical, or both, you must look at the capacity of that person to change. It is possible for some people to change with hard work, but only if they have a sincere desire and ability to acknowledge what is out of order in themselves. This requires a capacity to extend themselves for the sake of others, to respect the importance of owning their behavior, and a willingness to take responsibility for changing it as needed. When trying to determine if someone is capable of change, it is important to gain an understanding of his or her nature, rather than judge based on recent actions or behavior. Just because someone behaves badly does not mean they are a bad person; people can change if they are willing and able to make the necessary alterations.

I am willing to forgive someone and give them another chance as long as they show true remorse for harming me, a willingness to take responsibility for their behavior, express an honest intention to do better, and prove to me that they are making the needed changes by behaving differently. However, if this person is psychologically compromised in a way that makes all of this impossible, this must be acknowledged and faced.

It is not realistic to expect someone who is seriously mentally ill to act within a capacity they may not possess. All it would do is cause pain, frustration, bitterness, and disappointment for all parties involved. Psychological and emotional illnesses have an order to their severity, an individual potential for improvement with treatment, and a potential for a cure.

The Order of Disorder

There are three types of mental illnesses that come under the categories of psychological or emotional illnesses: psychotic disorders, personality disorders, and anxiety disorders. The following descriptions list the most drastic disorders with a relatively poor potential for improvement to the least drastic disorders with a relatively good potential for improvement. I call this list "the order of disorder."

1) Psychotic Disorders

The most serious mental illnesses fall under the category of psychological illness called Psychotic Disorders. Psychotic people are extremely difficult to treat and require a lifetime of care, including antipsychotic drugs that can yield little or no improvement. A person with a Psychotic Disorder suffers from psychosis, an aspect of psychological illness that is marked by delusions, hallucinations, incoherence, and an overall distorted perception of reality, such as in the cases of schizophrenia or mania. Mental hospitals are full of these tragic, suffering souls. The prognosis for improvement or cure in this group is very poor.

2) Personality Disorders (Ego-Syntonic)

The second most serious mental illnesses fall under the category of psychological illness, called Personality Disorders, which contains ten prominent conditions. Personality disorders are generally referred to as "ego-syntonic," when the disorder is marbleized throughout the entire personality and the sufferer believes that the drama, self-absorption, and other traits characterized by their condition are in fact reasonable responses to the way the world is treating them. This makes them hard patients to treat and cure. Anti-psychotic drugs can alleviate some of the stress of the most drastic cases and can motivate some patients to take on the harder work of therapy, where they can learn to modify and control their behavior.

These disorders are grouped into three distinct "subcategories" and are listed below from most drastic to least drastic. They are called the dramatic cluster, the anxious cluster, and the odd cluster.

- The first and most drastic of these subcategories is the "dramatic cluster." Of these, the best known are the Borderline, noted for their mellow-drama, the Antisocial, noted for being disruptive, the Narcissist, noted for their self-absorption, and the Histrionics, noted for making too much of things. These are the most toxic and destructive types of personality disorders and commonly occur in conjunction with other disorders

- The second is the "anxious cluster." These disorders include the straightforwardly named Dependent Personality (the Codependent), the Socially Withdrawn, the Avoidant Personality, and the rigid, rule-bound Obsessive-Compulsive Personality (entirely different from the anxiety condition called Obsessive-Compulsive Disorder).
- The third and least drastic group is the "odd cluster." These include the paranoid and schizoid personalities. The schizoid types have problems forming relationships and interpreting social cues. They are "lone wolves" (the classic recluse) that may also suffer from delusions, skating along the edge of real schizophrenia.

An increase in family fragmentation and dysfunction in our society is producing more cases of personality disorder than ever before. As much as nine percent of the general population is now thought to be suffering from some kind of personality disorder. As much as 20% of all mental health hospitalizations may be resultant of these conditions.

Studies show that after two years of therapy, 40% of patients suffering from the less drastic personality disorders show improvement, leaving 60% with the more drastic disorders who continue suffering and believing the lie the disorder tells them; that there is nothing wrong with them. They can eventually become more flexible and resilient but are not likely to stick with therapy. The prognosis for a cure in this group is poor.

3) Anxiety Disorders (Ego-Dystonic)

The third and least serious mental illnesses fall under the category of emotional illnesses called Anxiety Disorders, which includes phobias, compulsive worrying, eating disorders, and depression, and are generally referred to as "ego dystonic" when the sufferer is able to acknowledge the problem and wants to do something about it. These types of conditions are thought of as having a pathological rind wrapped around an intact core. Peel away the layers of the rind through talk therapy and/or melt them away with drugs and the problem has a good chance of abating.

These are neurotic disorders and can be treated with the greatest ease and success with hard work and dedication. Neuroses such as these can be completely cured in as little as six months to two years. Recovery usually requires a correction in the person's belief system and the replacement of an outdated map of life by creating a completely new one in order for the patient to be cured.

With the help of a good therapist, it will be up to you to determine which category the person or persons harming you may falls into. It will also be your responsibility to make a self-diagnosis according to what you learn about your dysfunctional family and yourself. If you want to heal yourself from chronic FMS and reclaim your life, you may have to face some hard facts. Sometimes facing these facts means leaving someone behind, giving them to God and giving yourself the chance you deserve to heal. If walking away from someone is what is necessary for you to heal then it is the choice you must make. We were not created to lay ourselves down as a sacrificial lamb to the pathologies of other human beings. It is our responsibility to use our God given free will in ways that will not allow this to happen by making the necessary choices that work to heal chronic FMS. This is your primary motivation for forgiveness: to heal and be well.

Motivation for Authentic Forgiveness

Forgiving is the kindest thing you can do for yourself because forgiveness heals wounds. The amazing grace of authentic forgiveness is more than the result of the rudimentary transaction of a transgressor making amends (remorse, apology, and promise to change). What about when amends is absent? Does a transgressor deserve to be forgiven if they show no remorse, give no subsequent apology, take no personal responsibility, and have no intention of making an effort to change?

The truth is, this does not morally concern you. This is between God and the transgressor. What does morally concern you is the act of authentic forgiveness: the deep, profound motion of the heart that initiates transcendence above anger. However, the act of forgiveness is not meant to absolve the transgressor of his or her personal responsibility. It is simply meant to cleanse the heart of the one doing the forgiving and release them from the scourge of festering anger.

To forgive someone who you do not feel deserves it is truly the kindest thing you can do for yourself. Holding grudges can actually cause the chronic release of toxic hormones, which do not help the healing process. Not only do these toxins aggravate FMS, they can make you sick independently of any other condition you may have. These hormones are released in conjunction with negative emotions, and should be avoided at all costs by someone already weakened by FMS. The behavior of someone else is not worth this kind of self-punishment. I heard someone say once that holding a grudge is like taking poison and waiting for other person to die. To forgive someone is to see forgiveness as a practical way to help you heal. It is also a profound way to love, nurture, and respect yourself, and only you have the power to do this.

Furthermore, the act of forgiveness does not mean going back for more abuse. It is very much the same as forgiving someone who has cheated you out of your life savings. You forgive them for your own sake, but you will never be foolish enough to trust them with your money again. If someone incapable of meeting your needs is harming you instead, then stop looking to them. It is wisdom to turn away and look to someone else, someone who is capable. Your first and foremost responsibility is to yourself, and you cannot take good care of yourself while allowing others to harm you.

I recently heard it said that wisdom and strength are not opposing forces. Wisdom comes from experience. Strength comes from self-love. Connecting to this reality will give you the courage to stay the course and not abandon yourself. Remember, when you no longer need anything from someone, detachment from him or her is made a lot easier and the freedom that accompanies it is extremely healing.

Tolstoy said in his book, *War And Peace*, "The most difficult thing is to love life even when you suffer, for to love life is to love God." So to love life and all it teaches, even through the suffering, is to love the self and the God within us all. Authentic forgiveness will release you from the past and ground you in the present to help you face the whole of your life, come what may. It will free you to live your life with courage, grace, and good cheer.

In the Holy Koran, Mohammed said, "He who seeketh approach me one cubit, I will seek to approach him two fathoms, and he who walketh towards me, I will run towards him, and he who cometh before me with the earth full of sins, but joineth no partner to me, I will come before him with an equal front of forgiveness." Free yourself from the shackles of non-forgiveness and forgive your transgressors for your own sake.

Forgiveness is Not The Same as Reconciliation

It is a common misconception that forgiveness is the same as reconciliation. The truth is, these two acts are entirely different in nature. Forgiveness deals solely with the past, while reconciliation concerns second chances and a desire for future change. Reconciliation is only possible when someone is willing to take responsibility for his or her behavior, express remorse, and make an honest attempt to do better.

When destructive behavior is brought to light, any honest attempt to own and correct such behavior will be demonstrated not by words, but by actions. If someone wants to reconcile but is not willing to change their behavior, then reconciliation is not possible.

No matter how badly you would like to reconcile with this person, if this is their response, there is nothing more you can do. When you are faced with an insincere apology, forgive the person for your own sake and do not give them the chance to repeat their fault. Wise men forgive, but only the fool forgets. Forgiveness in this instance simply means that you love yourself enough not to allow what happened in the past cause you to become frozen there, and will allow you to go on with your life unburdened by the past.

Forgiving the repentant or unrepentant transgressor means you realize it is their responsibility to correct their destructive behavior, and not your responsibility to adapt to it. When others are not capable of correcting their behavior, have compassion for them but stay detached and keep your distance. Even though you have forgiven, there are still going to be people and places you may always need to stay away from.

Furthermore, understanding bad behavior does not excuse it. It merely equips you to make accurate assessments for health and safety. By understanding the poor decisions of others, you can learn how to distance yourself from their adverse consequences and how to avoid making the same mistakes in your own life. Even if you understand why someone is behaving as they are, do not disregard poor behavior or make excuses for it.

In conclusion, forgive and reconcile when it is possible and equitable to do so. However, when you are faced with an unrepentant major offender or chronic abuser, choosing to squander your most precious personal resources (your time and your life force energy) by trying to reach someone who cannot understand you is more than foolish. It is martyrdom.

We were not given the gift of life to martyr ourselves to the incapacities of others. We are here to relish this precious gift by honoring and protecting ourselves from harm, discovering the meaning of our lives, fulfilling our potential for happiness, and finding our place in the world. When we are faced with a destructive relationship that proves hopeless, we must forgive and move on.

The Dark Night of The Soul

The awakening of the soul is the path of self-discovery. It is the journey of the spirit passing through a labyrinth of pain, grief, and purgation. In a spiritual classic, written by the famous Spanish Catholic mystic Saint John of the Cross, it is said, "Into this dark night souls begin to enter when God draws them forth from the state of beginners which is the state of those that meditate... and likewise how much these beginners in the virtues lack." He goes on to say, "Although we may tarry here for a time, it will not be longer than is necessary so that we may go on to speak of this dark night. And it will also be seen how many blessings the dark night of which we shall afterwards treat brings with us, since it cleanses the soul and purifies it from these imperfections." He describes these "beginners imperfections" as the seven capital sins: pride, avarice, luxury, wrath, gluttony, envy, and sloth.

Another description of the dark night of the soul is about the spiritual value of the suffering and the stripping away of all that we have ever believed in. Taking away all that we have relied on in the past begins the process of unfolding the true self by falling into the "abyss," where the battle is waged between our commitment to ourselves and our innate human laziness. As a test of our truest character, this process is an inevitable part of our human experience, something we all have in common, and something that is unavoidable. This journey to self-knowing is always referred to in spiritual terms, called a spiritual crisis, spiritual emergency, or spiritual, divine, or holy madness.

Buddha says, "The dharma of self-knowing is the simplest thing in the world, and the most difficult thing in the world." It is also the most valuable thing in the world. To know thyself is to know God. To know God is to know love, and love is the greatest force on earth.

Chapter Four
Understanding Chronic Fibromyalgia

Chronic fibromyalgia syndrome (FMS) is a descriptive name for a long-term condition of the body involving the central nervous system, soft tissue, and pain. The word "chronic" means having a particular long-term condition that causes long-term changes in the body. The term fibromyalgia is made up of the Greek root *fibro*, referring to fibrous or scar tissue. Myalgia is made up of the Greek root *myo*, meaning muscle, and *algia*, meaning a painful condition. Put them all together and they mean a long-term condition of fibrous and muscle tissue pain. The word syndrome refers to a group of symptoms that, together, characterize a specific disease or disorder. Although the term chronic fibromyalgia syndrome describes a prevalent part of this disease (the tissue pain), it is not really broad enough to represent the condition in its entirety.

Another term often used alone or in conjunction with chronic FMS is chronic fatigue syndrome. The word fatigue means a temporary state of extreme weakness or tiredness with an inability of an organ or part, such as a muscle or nerve cell, to respond to a stimulus and function normally following continuous activity or stimulation. Like the term chronic fibromyalgia syndrome, the term chronic fatigue syndrome is a descriptive term that addresses only a part of the condition and falls short of accurately accounting for every aspect of the disorder.

A comprehensive overview of chronic fibromyalgia syndrome reveals it as a state of chronic, massive energy deficit or dysenergism, a lack of adequate energy/ATP production by the body on a cellular level. Dysenergism is caused by massively distorted signals to and from the brain that result in an overly stimulated and hyper-sensitized central nervous system (CNS). The system-wide biological imbalances and malfunctions caused by this deadly combination of chronic dysenergism, distorted brain signals, and an overly stimulated and hyper-sensitized CNS are catastrophic. Currently these combined effects are called chronic fibromyalgia syndrome/chronic fatigue syndrome.

The History of Chronic FMS

As early as 1843, Dr. Robert Friedrich Froriep described, in text, a medical condition he called "rheumatism with painful hard places that can be felt in various locations on the body," and "tender areas in muscles that felt like a cord associated with rheumatic complaints." This is considered to be the first known description of chronic FMS in modern medical texts. In 1904, Sir William Gowers of University College Hospital in London, England began a study of his own lumbago, initially calling it *fibrositis.*

In 1993, New Year's Day, the World Health Organization (WHO) declared FMS a syndrome and the most common cause of wide spread muscle pain. WHO incorporated an American College of Rheumatology 1990 definition, citing as criteria 18 "tender points" symmetrically located throughout the human body. Today, the gold standard for diagnosing chronic FMS is the presence of muscle pain and involvement of at least 11 out of these 18 tender points.

WHO also said, "Fibromyalgia is part of a wider syndrome encompassing headaches, irritable bladder, dysmenorrhea, cold sensitivity, Reynaud's phenomenon, restless legs, atypical patterns of numbness and tingling, exercise intolerance and complaints of weakness and depression."

Jacob Teitelbaum, MD, medical director of Maryland's Annapolis Center for Effective CHF/FMS Therapy, states, "FMS patients seem to have genetic differences in the way their hypothalamus, pituitary and adrenal regulation handles stress. As a result the muscles end up short of energy and in pain." However, the consequences of chronic energy deficit are much more than muscle and connective tissue pain.

I read a lovely quote once about the dark night of the soul that went something like this, "In falling into the abyss, within the hole of the dark night of failure and discouragement, the stars shine brightly, and the darker the night, the brighter the stars. Every one of us has special gifts and can make a difference. The trouble is people sometimes fall into the darkness and stay there. You must find and follow your own star. It will lead you out of the darkness." Finding and following your star is finding and listening to your inner guide. It will lead you out of the abyss of chronic FMS and set you on the path toward regained health; however, you will not be able to navigate this path if you do not understand your condition.

In 2002, a homeopathic doctor gave me an interesting, lesser-known description of chronic fibromyalgia syndrome. He called the condition, "neuromuscular facilitation with the resting potential set too high." Facilitation in this context means a decrease in the resistance to a nerve impulse in a neural pathway brought about by prior or repeated stimulation, such as exercise.

This decrease in resistance means that the normal controls that exist for a nerve impulse are malfunctioning, allowing an inappropriately high amount of nerve impulses to occur and remain in the pathway. This results in the resting potential, or the state of a muscle when it is not in action, being reset at a level higher than that of a state of rest. These uncontrolled nerve impulses are called *distortion signals.*

The doctor explained that, in my condition, a distortion signal coming from the part of the brain called the hypothalamus was causing a distortion, or over-firing, of the nerves along the neural pathways, resulting in the resting potential of the muscles to be set too high. When the resting potential is set too high, muscles are prevented from being completely at rest at a level of non-action. As a result, the muscles and connective tissues remain chronically tense.

The doctor also called my condition myofascial pain syndrome, which is the shortening of connective and muscle tissue due to chronic tension, and said I did not have fibromyalgia. It is not uncommon for someone with chronic FMS to receive this kind of partial and incorrect diagnosis. Myofascial pain syndrome is a symptom of chronic FMS.

His homeopathic term for chronic FMS describes the condition in a little more detail than those offered by regular medicine; however, it still does not entirely account for all of the symptoms that fall under the large umbrella of fibromyalgia. This homeopathic term also contains the theory of distortion signals coming from the brain and asserts that these out-of-control, hyper-charged, distorted nerve impulses are caused by a physical or psychological trauma or stress, which we will explore in more detail later in the book.

Often called the "invisible disability," chronic FMS is still being referred to by a few uninformed medical professionals as a catchall name for a "collection of bizarre symptoms shared by a group of neurotic women." An article in the October 2006 issue of *Alternative Medicine Magazine* stated that chronic FMS affects about two percent of all Americans (two percent of currently 500 million), and accounts for up to thirty percent of all rheumatology medical consultations.

The 2009 online statistics from "Fibromyalgia Statistics" state that there are over 90 million reported FMS cases worldwide, and over ten million of these are in the United States. These cases represent a $12 - $14 billion annual cost for treatment and a one to two percent annual loss of productivity. Although we have seen this illness begin in patients as early as age four and as late as seventy four, it mainly affects women between the ages of 35 and 55, occurring ten times more frequently in women than men.

Interestingly, because the National FMS Research Association stated that 90% of all fibromyalgia patients are women, many believe that, genetically, at least one FMS gene is carried on the female "X" chromosome. However, due to the wide spread age onset, FMS is impossible to explain with only one inherited gene. Common sense can say this statistic could simply be explained by the fact that men are generally built physically stronger than women and thus have stronger musculature in their neck, shoulders and back. They are therefore less vulnerable to injuries to the neck and spine that trigger chronic FMS. Sometimes there really can be a simple explanation for an otherwise "unexplained phenomenon" based on common sense

It Takes Energy To Run The Body

Energy is one of the most important components of a healthy body. It runs our entire body and brain functions, including:

- The heart, for pumping steady blood.
- The liver to detoxify the blood and produce insulin, along with other metabolic functions.
- The spleen that, among other things, destroys old red blood cells and forms lymphocytes for fighting infection and cancer.
- The lymphatic system, which produces and houses lymphocytes and filters microorganisms and other unwanted particles from lymph fluids.
- The endocrine glandular system, which secretes lymph or hormones directly into the blood from the thyroid, pituitary, pineal, and adrenal glands.
- The thymus gland, located at the base of the skull, which develops the cells of the immune system, particularly T-cells, a type of lymphocyte (white blood cell) that is crucial in fighting viral infections and cancer.
- The digestive system: the stomach that breaks down food, the intestines that absorb the food nutrients, and the colon and anus that regulate and dispose of waste materials.
- The urinary tract system, including the kidneys that filter liquid waste from the blood, excreting it as urine through the bladder.
- The reproductive system.
- The brain, to process data and to form new neural pathways to store, recall, and analyze the data and to maintain clarity and fluidity in thought and verbal expressions. In addition, the brain runs the autonomic nervous system, which regulates involuntary functions, such as heart beat and glandular secretions.

Without enough energy, none of these function can maintain a healthy balance. Chronic FMS is a paradox that combines extreme dysenergism (inadequate energy/ATP production in the cells) with the distortion and/or over-firing of bio-chemical impulses and signals to and from the brain. These impulses and signals travel from the brain into the body through the CNS along complex nerve pathways or wires.

Regulatory Centers of The Hypothalamus

The most critical organ the body depends upon for overall functioning is the hypothalamus. It is located in the mid-back of the brain and uses the most energy for its size than any other organ. A shortfall of energy in the body is sure to cause this organ to malfunction and jump off line first. This can create enormous consequences, as this small organ is the body's chief watchdog. Through its regulatory centers, the hypothalamus guards and regulates key biological functions that we depend on. The regulatory centers inside the hypothalamus control the following biological functions:

- Sleep cycle
- Day/night cycle
- Body temperature
- Blood pressure and circulation
- Thirst and fluid retention
- Appetite and fullness
- Metabolism
- Hormone secretions
- Balancing of cerebral neurotransmitters in the sympathetic and parasympathetic nervous systems
- Primal emotions

Like the hippocampus, anther major function of the hypothalamus in conjunction with the limbic system around its edge, is the storage of our memories. Since our memories consist of both positive and negative events, in theory the hypothalamus can also store the positive and negative emotional charge that coincides with these impressions. The limbic system, an interconnected system of brain nuclei, is associated with basic needs and emotions such as hunger, pain, pleasure, satisfaction, sex drive, and instinctive motivation.

The hypothalamus plays a major role in handling stress and maintaining health and balance throughout the body, and its malfunction can decrease the body's protective abilities dramatically. The result is a cascade of biological system imbalances and malfunctions, exacerbated by the massive dysenergism/energy deficit and chronic fatigue inherent in chronic fibromyalgia syndrome.

General Diagnostic Criteria

The National FMS Research Association states that there are over ten million people in the United States and 90 million people worldwide known to suffer from FMS. However, this condition is so often misdiagnosed or unreported, the actual number of cases is most likely much higher. FMS is commonly diagnosed as myofascial pain syndrome, chronic fatigue syndrome, or rheumatoid arthritis. Other diagnostic terms used ending in "itis" (meaning inflammation) are fibrositis and fibromyocitis. These terms are no longer used because it is now believed that there is no inflammation in chronic fibromyalgia syndrome, although it may occur at its onset.

Chronic fibromyalgia manifests itself in a large variety of what appear to be unrelated symptoms in an almost endless number of combinations, and sometimes the lines between individual symptoms become blurred. There are no known clinical tests that can diagnose FMS with any degree of certainty. Because of these facts and a common unfamiliarity of this syndrome among today's medical professionals, it often takes a long time to obtain a proper diagnosis.

Since it manifests so widely throughout the body, another problem in diagnosing FMS is that one or more symptoms can be "mis-grouped," causing the condition to appear to be something else. The term FMS is actually a large umbrella over a long list of manifested symptoms. Chronic FMS can even be viewed a symptom itself, a symptom of its cause. This concept still eludes much of the professional medical community. However, awareness about fibromyalgia is growing, along with the medical professional's profound sense of frustration about treating FMS successfully.

Making FMS even more difficult to properly diagnose is the fact that not every fibromyalgia patient suffers from every symptom that falls under the FMS umbrella. It is the rule and not the exception that each FMS patient suffers from their own individual combination of symptoms, although there are certain symptoms that most FMS patients experience at any stage of the disease. FMS is unique in that it affects so many parts of the body, and one patient's primary complaint can be different from another's.

The predominant group of symptoms, or the primary complaint each patient experiences at the time of diagnosis, depends upon such factors as genetic predispositions, the stage of their FMS, the severity of their condition, and the length of time the patient has been ill. Patients in the early stages may not develop symptoms they may develop later on when FMS becomes "full blown."

Sometimes the condition burdensomely lumbers along, affecting overall general health for many years in ways that are not severe enough to identify a disabling or primary complaint. Sometimes symptoms develop gradually, increasing in intensity over time. In addition, they can be triggered or worsened by different factors, including compounding injury, trauma, depression, anxiety, stress, lack of exercise, overexertion, lack of sleep, grief, extremes of temperature and/or humidity, and infectious disease.

The condition can also rapidly spiral into "full blown" FMS and manifest with more than one disabling or *"loud"* symptoms. The course of FMS is unpredictable and not all cases become chronic or full blown; some cases clear up on their own over time, while some seem transitory and go through cycles of "flare-ups" alternating with periods of apparent remission. However, the majority of FMS cases are so severe that symptoms interfere with daily life, completely disabling a significant number of these patients.

An accurate diagnosis may become obstructed when a patient seeks help from a specialist in the field of their primary complaint. Specialists are used to analyzing their patients through the lens of his or her own specialty and may not look to causes that may be beyond their field of expertise. Because of this, doctors can mistakenly treat the patient's primary complaint as the entire disease, overlooking the fact that there is a much larger problem. FMS by nature is "a complex of symptoms" often experienced at different stages, which must be seen as the many manifestations of fibromyalgia. Understanding this helps reduce the time it takes to reach a proper diagnosis.

Some doctors experience a lot of confusion and frustration when evaluating a fibromyalgia patient. This "unseen disability" is a gigantic mystery in the modern world of conventional medicine. Without a clearly established cause, cure, or treatment, FMS is still a mystery to many in the conventional health care profession.

Some doctors will not even attempt treating a patient that has been diagnosed with FMS. One of these is Dr. Andrew Weil, the acclaimed "guru of alternative medicine," author of several popular healing books, repeat speaker on the PBS lecture circuit, and founder of his own alternative medical clinic in Scottsdale, Arizona. I heard him say on CNN's *Larry King Live* in a November 10th, 2004 interview, "We won't take a patient with fibromyalgia in our Arizona clinic. We won't treat them because its just too frustrating and we don't know what to do with them."

I understand this condition may be very confusing and frustrating for doctors, but I guarantee it is much more so for FMS patients. While doctors can refer patients to other medical specialists, the patients are stuck dealing with the disease while the doctors try to find the correct diagnosis.

FMS can take up to 30 years to present itself in a major way. This is why I believe the most sensible and expedient way for a doctor to go about evaluating a potential fibromyalgia patient is to allow enough time during their initial consultation to hear the patient's full medical history as far back as the patient can remember, including all injuries, traumas, and illnesses.

During the process of identifying a primary FMS complaint there is sure to be a long and confusing list of seemingly unrelated secondary symptoms. Just as important as forming a clear picture of the patient's history is bringing to light all the stress factors involved throughout the patient's life, past and present in addition to the stress of FMS.

In addition to looking for fatigue and lack of energy in FMS, other common symptoms are insomnia, sleep disturbance, and a dizziness that goes hand in hand with a cognitive impairment known as "fibro-fog." Fibro-fog includes the inability to think clearly, retain information, remember recent events, and coherently express thoughts.

Widespread muscle pain and tender points are common. As I mentioned earlier, the "tender point test," in relation to FMS, requires at least 11 of a possible 18 tender points on the body to be sensitive to mild pressure or touch. This sensitivity may be represented by pain or soreness, and if at least 11 spots are present along with the above symptoms, it is safe to say that fibromyalgia is present.

With the multitude of symptoms that manifest in this condition, and the countless combinations in which they may appear, an old axiom holds that, "When all other contingencies fail, that which remains, however improbable, must be the truth." Because there are so many seemingly unrelated symptoms and disorders that fall under the chronic FMS umbrella, the next section concentrates on the most known to date.

Specific Symptomatology of FMS

The most common symptoms associated with FMS are: chronic wide spread body pain (90% - 100% of patients); at least 11 out of 18 tender points (90% - 100%); chronic fatigue (90% - 100%); cognitive impairment or fibro-fog (70% - 90%); sleep disturbances (70% - 90%); dysmenorhea or painful menstruation (70% - 90%); and irritable bowel syndrome (50% - 70%).

Other chronic symptoms manifesting in FMS are: myofascial pain syndrome; body wide muscle twitching and fluttering; muscle spasms in the form of ropes, bundles, knots, and bands; muscle sensations, including various kinds of pain, such as a feeling of ground glass between the muscle layers, a raw, gnawing, or tearing feeling in the muscles, and burning, aching, or soreness of muscles; and restless leg syndrome.

Further chronic symptoms include: candidiasis; interstitial cystitis; dysuria (difficult urination); vulvar pain syndrome (vulvodynia); migraine syndrome; indigestion; peptic ulcer disease; nausea; excessive gas; constipation; diarrhea; esophageal spasms (difficulty swallowing); poor circulation; constantly being cold; constantly being hot; sweating; burning skin; buzzing skin; numbness; anxiety and depression; loss of memory; blurred vision; dry eye syndrome; eye irritation or burning with a discharge of stinging tears; dizziness and vertigo arising from the middle ear; excessive nasal congestion; and mucus in the throat.

The list of chronic symptoms goes on: sinusitis; bronchitis; heart palpitations; mitral valve prolapse; TMJ (temporomandibular joint syndrome); rheumatic disorder; itchy, dry, or flaky skin; brittle and flaky nails; dry or brittle hair; excess tooth tarter; strange mouth sensations (metallic, dry, or scalded feeling); carbohydrate craving; sugar craving; salt craving; sensitivities to chemicals, light, sound, and odors; tinnitis (ringing, buzzing, or throbbing sounds in the inner ear); and excessive ear wax production.

This bizarre "incurable" illness with its "unknown etiology" and its unique cycles of good and bad days has one constant unmitigated factor: years and years of unceasing pain and misery unlike any other disease on the planet.

To further explain the various ways chronic fibromyalgia symptoms manifest within a number of biological systems, I will categorize these systems in six general groups or biological systems.

The Biological Systems Affected By FMS

1) Central Nervous System

The central nervous system is where chronic FMS lives, breathes, and multiplies. When the central nervous system goes haywire, everything else goes to hell. This is what causes the myriad of symptoms listed above. The signals from the brain to the body regulating its systems and functions, and the signals from the body to the brain delivering messages for it to process and respond to, become completely distorted in chronic FMS. The brain cannot make heads or tails of these crisscrossing signals.

The resulting chronic fatigue/dysenergism makes it even harder for the brain to operate properly. Thinking, feeling, sensing, reacting, responding, evaluating, balancing, and overall function become distorted, dulled, confused, off, underactive, hyperactive, hypersensitive, etc. in numerous ways. When brain signals are distorted they become too weak or too strong all at the wrong times, and the entire body is affected.

2) Musculoskeletal System

The musculoskeletal system is affected by the most devastating symptoms manifested in this condition: intense, widespread, chronic pain. Many doctors will not believe your testimony of this unseen symptom. The only hint of an indication of this neuromuscular pain being real is a test called a reflex test, where the doctor takes a rubber mallet and taps lightly on certain areas around the joints, typically the knee. In fibromyalgia, the central nervous system is so hypersensitive that the reflex test results are off the charts "without any apparent reason." Other than this test and the tender points test, the doctor just has to believe what you tell him about your symptoms.

When a doctor does not believe you it can be devastating. I had one doctor say to me once, "Why don't you go out and take a walk in the mall and get your mind off your problems?" This was at a time when I was in so much pain that I had been bed-ridden for nearly a year and could barely walk from my bed into the bathroom. A psychiatrist who was doing a personality evaluation concluded that I was a "hysterical hypochondriac whose emotional problems will continue to plague her marriage until she resolves them." Neither of these doctors understood or believed the extremity of my pain.

This type of treatment is medical abuse. If your doctor does not believe you when you tell him what is wrong and what you are feeling, then keep looking until you find a doctor who is knowledgeable about FMS. Sometimes doctors try to find other reasons for your symptoms when they do not understand your condition. This can lead to your pain being blamed on emotional stress or an overactive imagination, and this is unacceptable. Do not let your pain be shrugged off as fiction; find a doctor who understands FMS and will be able to make your life better. There are doctors who will listen to you, believe you, diagnose you properly, and do everything they can to help you within the limits of their profession, and if they are stumped, they will say so. I went through fifteen doctors in twelve years before I received an accurate diagnosis, so I understand how stressful finding the right doctor can be; however, the process is worth the stress if you can find a doctor you can rely on.

Knowledge about fibromyalgia is becoming more prevalent today than ever before and is increasing all the time, but the medical profession has a long way to go before they understand it fully. Because fibromyalgia is not completely understood, most medical doctors rely heavily on prescription drugs to try to reduce the pain experienced by their patients. I hope that, in reading this, you will learn how to treat your fibromyalgia in healthier ways, and will share this knowledge and experience with your doctor.

Maybe in 20 years society will view our current medical approaches for treating chronic illness like we now view medical methods employed 100 years ago, when doctors would bleed their patients who had infectious diseases. These archaic beliefs can be attributed to a lack of knowledge, technology and resources. As our knowledge and technology improves, our medical profession will be better equipped to handle the pain of fibromyalgia. Until then, we must look to other options for curing this disease.

There are many types of chronic widespread pain. These types of pain can be constant or intermittent, severe or mild, stationary or transient, can come and go in cycles, and can move around the body by taking up residence in different areas of the body at different times. There are also many kinds of pain that can come in an endless number of combinations. These kinds of pain are often referred to as: sharp; dull; stinging; burning; tingling; deep; surface; aching; gnawing; shooting; stabbing; prickly; electric impulses that feel like "electric worms"; sore; tender; grabbing; gripping; cramping; tight or stiff tendons, ligaments, and muscles; and even a numbness in the face and extremities that is usually caused by constricted structures pressing on nearby nerves. Understanding the terms for the type and kind of pain you are experiencing will not only help your doctor understand you, it will help you understand yourself and feel a little less confused, and a lot more sane.

Restless Leg Syndrome

Restless Leg Syndrome (RLS) is a very painful symptom manifested in the musculoskeletal system. RLS is caused by cycles of electrical impulses that surge through the muscles of the legs cause jerking, twitching, and spasms, and it almost always occurs when you lie back or lie down to rest or sleep. The cycles of these symptoms can be very painful, making it impossible to get comfortable, to rest, or go to sleep. RLS pain heightens pain from other FMS symptoms by not allowing you to sleep. This forces you to experience extreme pain and exhaustion, which is a miserable feeling.

The electrical impulses that surge through the legs occur in cycles or intervals that can last up to thirty or forty seconds, with only a few seconds of rest between cycles. These surges can involve an entire leg or one side of a body, or they can happen in both legs and involve both sides of the body at the same time. The nerve impulses released into the legs through these surges seem to be impulses that have been blocked by tension in the soft tissue surrounding key points along neural pathways. This prevents nerve impulses from traveling normally along what Chinese medicine calls "meridians."

My theory, which I composed after experiencing restless leg syndrome in both legs for many years, is that blocked, congested energy builds up at an area of soft tissue constriction in the hips, back, or shoulders until the congestion of energy reaches a critical level. This energy then explodes into the nervous system and through the legs or other parts of the body, causing the painful twitching and spasms. This explosive release temporarily alleviates the energy congestion that quickly builds up again, and the cycle is repeated and can continue for hours or until you go to sleep.

I have experienced restless leg symptoms in one leg at times and in both legs at other times. It has even expanded to include my shoulders and spine and my entire body. Sometimes just rolling over on one side, bending into a fetal position, and wrapping my arms around my shins can shut it off. If this does not work, you can try to get relief by doing some gentle stretching of tightest areas, if you can, taking a hot bath in Epson salts. If all else fails, taking a gentle sleep aid, such as Valerian Root, Melatonin, L-Theonine, or half doses of Excedrin PM or Tylenol PM. In my experience stretching the tight areas works best, but I have at some point resorted to each of these methods.

When stretching, a yoga position called *"child's pose"* has worked very well for me when I had the most trouble. To do the child's pose, roll over and raise up onto your hands and knees, with hands shoulder width apart and knees a little wider than hip width apart. Bring your big toes together and then slowly sit back and place your hips on or over your heals with the bottom of your feet toward the ceiling. Lower your buttocks down as close to your heals as is comfortable, lay your chest down on a pillow between your thighs and place your forehead on the bed between your arms. You can use a pillow to support your forehead, too, if you cannot bend your neck far enough to touch the bed, but keep your head and neck straight with the spine.

Keep your hands in their original positions, rest your arms down on the bed, and relax there for as long as the pose provides relief, about five to ten minutes if you can. Keep your focus on relaxing into the pose and concentrate on easy, steady breathing through the nose with your tongue relaxed on the floor of your mouth and an open, "ah" shaped throat. If your arms feel too uncomfortable lying above your head, move them down to your side with the palms rotated toward the ceiling. If the constriction in the tissues around key nerves causing your restless legs is in your back, shoulders, or hips, this stretch will relieve it enough to stop the energy congestion and you should be able to roll over and go to sleep.

Temporomandibular Joint Syndrome

Temporomandibular Joint Syndrome (TMJ) involves muscles and tendons around the jaw joint that connect the temporal bone (the bone that forms the side of the skull) with the mandible (the jawbone). This condition is estimated to affect upwards of ten million Americans, the same estimated amount of people with FMS! Stress and tension in the ligaments and tendons around the joint of the jaw is the most common underlying cause. TMJ can be caused by an Atlas subluxation, whiplash, or a hard blow to the jaw or chin. Even poor posture can also affect the alignment of the jaw.

The jaw joint is embedded in an intricate web of nerves and muscles along the side of the face and neck, and when tension or trauma presses on these nerves it can cause a variety of problems. Primarily, the cartilage disc that cushions the joint may become displaced or wear out, causing the bones of the temporomandibular joint to rub against each other instead of gliding smoothly past one another. In many cases, this misalignment of the jaw and teeth can prevent smooth operation of the joint.

Aside from causing difficulty chewing, the excruciating pain that can be experienced in the joints and muscles of the jaw can radiate into the face, head, neck, and shoulders. This pain can be so severe it can completely disable a person, and can even expand from the affected area to radiate throughout much of the body. This is called an expansion or widening of pain receptor fields, or "receptor field enlargement." TMJ can also affect the jaw by causing difficulty in fully opening the joint.

During chewing or joint movement, you may hear clicking, popping, and grinding noises. TMJ can cause migraine strength headaches, dizziness, toothaches, a feeling of pain and pressure behind the eyes, pain and ringing in the ears, and difficulty opening and closing the jaw normally. The force of chewing normally creates a tremendous pressure on the nerves and muscles of the jaw and can aggravate TMJ, as does gritting the teeth, grinding the teeth during the night, or chewing gum. Like FMS, TMJ is made much worse with stress. Often there were times when the stress of my FMS was so heavy, I would get what I called a

TMJ migraine headache, which always began at the base of my skull behind my right ear and jaw. TMJ can affect one or both sides of the jaw, but mine was only in the right jaw, as the great majority of my FMS symptoms were right-sided. Although my TMJ was constant for 30 years, it was never disabling in itself. The popping and stabbing pain occasionally prevented me from chewing, but it usually abated.

My TMJ no longer bothers me unless I am under large amounts of stress, and it no longer causes migraine headaches. I found quick relief from TMJ headaches with two over the counter migraine formula tablets containing acetaminophen, aspirin, and caffeine. The best approach for me was to relax and unlock the jaw joint, relax my tongue onto the floor of my mouth, not to open my mouth too wide, and concentrate of my breathing for ten to fifteen minutes. As this is a very good habit to form for overall relaxation, it also relaxed the stress on the jaw and lessened the pain.

A wonderful book entitled *Prescriptions for Natural Healing,* written by Phyllis A. Balch, CNC, and James F. Balch, MD, offers plenty of nutritional suggestions to supplement your diet along with a TMJ self-test to determine if your jaw may be misaligned. First, you put the tip of your forefingers in your ears and then you open and close your jaw slowly and carefully. If at any point you hear a popping, clicking, or grinding noise your jaw may be out of alignment.

Specialists in TMJ can diagnose and treat a misalignment of the jaw and also provide prosthetic mouthpieces to wear at night to put space between the upper and lower molars, which helps relax the jaw and prevent teeth grinding while you sleep. If you consult a specialist, make sure he or she knows that you have FMS. I suggest seeing a cervical chiropractor first to check for an Atlas misalignment, the most common cause of TMJ.

With TMJ you should also avoid highly processed foods, such as sugar, white flour, pasta, potatoes, junk food, and soda. Stress management and relaxation techniques are essential, and when combined with mild heat applied to the jaw pain area, may relax tense joint muscles. Try to avoid muscle relaxants, as their side effects are often not worth their benefits. Valerian root capsules taken at bedtime will help relax your muscles, as well as help you get to sleep. Take Valerian root two weeks on and two weeks off or every other night to avoid developing a resistance to it. When you sleep, try to sleep on your back as much as you can to rest your neck, shoulders and back muscles so they remain as relaxed as possible.

Tender Points

The eighteen tender points of chronic fibromyalgia are considered to be the disease's most distinctive feature, and the only one that differentiates it from similar conditions. These tender points are also called trigger points and tend to group symmetrically around the body near muscles, tendons, and ligaments, and appear around the neck, shoulders, chest, knees, elbows, and hips.

Specific tender point locations are: the lower vertebra of the neck; at the insertions of the second rib; the upper part of the thigh bone; in the middle of the knee joint; in muscles connected to the base of the skull; in muscles of the neck and upper back; in muscles of the mid-back; on the side of the elbows; and in the upper and outer muscles of the buttocks. The pain or tenderness in these tender points can be intermittent or constant, can move from one area of the body to another, and can vary from day to day.

Tender points have fascinated doctors and chronic fibromyalgia patients alike since the 1840's, when doctors referred to them in rheumatic patients as "painful hard places." In chronic fibromyalgia, at least 11 out of the possible 18 tender points in predetermined sites are sore or painful to the touch. The sensitivity of these points can vary, and they can be relatively small or involve entire muscle bundles that seem swollen and very painful. These tender points have become known among many fibromyalgics as the "lumps and bumps" of fibromyalgia.

3) Cerebrum and Cerebellum

Parts of the brain that can be severely affected are the cerebrum and the cerebellum. These parts of the brain are also home to cognitive impairment, which is known as fibro-fog (the inability to concentrate and sporadic memory loss). In some FMS patients, these symptoms can be primary for an undetermined period of time before eventually developing a chronic widespread pain syndrome. However, most patients are foggy, exhausted and in pain.

Many patients feel their fibro-fog has an equally negative impact on their lives as their pain, and patients with an extremely high pain threshold consider their cognitive impairment and fatigue to be their primary complaint. Chronic fibromyalgia syndrome and chronic fatigue syndrome were once believe to be separate conditions; however, due to the vast overlap of symptoms, it is now widely understood that they are indeed the same malady. In fact, chronic fatigue syndrome is now considered to be an FMS symptom.

The cerebrum is the front part of the brain and is divided into two symmetrical halves, or cerebral hemispheres. Its primary function involves activities including reasoning, learning, sensory perception, and emotional responses. The cerebellum, located behind the cerebrum, is also divided into two symmetrical hemispheres connected by a thin central region. Its main function is to control and coordinate muscular activity and maintain balance. When the dysenergism (lack of adequate energy production on a cellular level) of fibromyalgia affects the brain, the manifested symptoms are wide.

Cerebral symptoms in chronic FMS include: waves of tsunami-like depression; anxiety; nervousness; irritability; unpredictable mood-swings; chronic, mind-numbing fatigue; sudden or chronic exhaustion; apathy; sleep disturbances (insomnia, frequently awakening during the night, nightmares, and non-restorative sleep); dizziness; loss of balance; blurred vision; and headaches, which can be as severe as migraines.

When wide spread pain is experienced, the severity of these cerebral symptoms seems to coincide in degree with the severity of the pain, and manifest together in mysterious "cycles." Factors such as stress, trauma, too much outside stimulation or distractions, and fatigue can exacerbate these mental disabilities just as these factors can exacerbate many other symptoms of fibromyalgia. When symptoms suddenly become worse and then subside, this is called a "flare-up."

Medicating chronic depression with antidepressants in the belief that depression causes fibromyalgia is an outdated approach. It is now well understood that depression is not the cause of FMS. Common sense dictates that anyone who lives with the pain and fatigue of chronic fibromyalgia would soon become depressed. In fact, studies show that FMS patients are no more depressed than another group of patients who live with chronic pain. Even a healthy person who is simply sleep deprived would soon become chronically depressed, exhausted, and would experience impairment in their mental functions.

Because both pain and depression are believed to share common neural receptors in the brain, the use of antidepressants has shown to be helpful in reducing depression while simultaneously helping to reduce physical pain in fibromyalgics. The main point here is that fibromyalgia is not a psychological illness, nor is it a "bizarre, changeable array of symptoms manifested in a large group of hysterical women." The idea of medicating FMS symptoms such as chronic fatigue, cognitive impairment/fibro-fog, and sleep disturbances with prescription sleep aids holds to the belief that falsely creating a more restorative sleep will eliminate these symptoms. This is also an erroneous approach. Frequent napping during the day helps relieve symptoms to a degree; however taking prescription sleep medications to help you sleep through the night can cause further problems.

For example, when you begin a prescription sleep aid you are generally given the lowest effective dose. Eventually, the body develops a resistance to this dose and a higher dose is needed, and so on. Furthermore, even the lowest dose can cause a "hangover," because sleep aids cause a slowing in cerebral thought connections that lasts into the next day. Also, the higher the dose of a sleep medication the more intense the hangover, creating a heavier feeling of mental fogginess overall. Add this to the deprivations of fibro-fog and you will probably decide you are waking up feeling worse, not better. This is not a helpful cycle to enter into and will not eliminate the symptoms of what I call chronic *"fibro-brain,"* which includes fatigue, fibro-fog, and sleep disturbances.

Sleep disturbances are a major problem and a serious concern for fibromyalgics. A recent publication of *Alternative Medicine Magazine* stated that 90% of FMS patients wake up multiple times during the night, and when they can sleep through most of the night it is not deep enough to be restorative and rejuvenating. There are several FMS symptoms that interrupt sleep, including irritable bowel, restless legs, and a condition called "nocturnal myoclonus," which simply means jerky muscles.

The resulting interrupted and non-restorative sleep is what scientists call *"disregulated sleep physiology,"* where the alpha rhythm disturbances that occur during the night prevent the deep sleep that is necessary to make growth hormones, create the biochemical energy (ATP = adenosine triphosphate) necessary to recharge your batteries, and heal the ravages of the day. It has been suggested that taking 200 milligrams at bedtime of the alternative sleep aid L-theanine can help you sleep soundly through the night without waking up groggy. You can also try the older alternative sleep aid Melatonin, about two or three milligrams at bedtime, not to exceed five milligrams. However, too much Melatonin can cause you to sleep too deeply, resulting in horrible nightmares in vivid technicolor. If you are too sensitive for even the lowest dose available, try cutting the pill in half.

Because an uninterrupted sleep cycle is so critical, if you must take a prescription sleep aid try to maintain as low a dose as possible. You can try alternating your prescription sleep-aid with other non-prescription alternatives, such as Valerian Root, Melatonin, L-Theonine, Tylenol PM, or Excedrin PM. Take these in moderation, too, for the same reasons. Note: be sure to check with your physician or homeopath for safety if you are taking any other medication or remedy.

Not taking your prescription sleep aid every night and alternating it with non-prescription sleep-aids will help prevent your body from developing a tolerance to the lowest doses you are trying. Also, remember to drink about six to eight eight-ounce glasses of water during the day to help flush medications from your body. Some FMS patients have experienced a disappearance of many symptoms when managing to get regular deep sleep, however their symptoms returned when they did not. Whatever you decide to try, do the very best you can to minimize your sleep-aid dependency, take as many naps as you need to, and never, ever push yourself too hard.

4) Digestive System

The digestive system also has its share of various system-wide problems. There are several gastrointestinal disorders that fall under the FMS umbrella. The most prominent of these is irritable bowel syndrome (IBS), also known as spastic colon. IBS includes symptoms such as painful excess gas and bloating, intestinal cramps, unpredictable attacks of diarrhea alternating with constipation, nausea, and gastric hyperacidity. Stress can easily worsen IBS, and even cause a severe attack.

The stress of FMS is already so much to cope with, it is vitally important to eliminate all other forms of unnecessary stress whenever possible, especially if you suffer from this particular FMS symptom. Making some major life-altering changes may eliminate major stressors, such as a marriage that has gone bad, a stressful job, or a toxic or chaotic living environment. Irritable bowel syndrome is serious and must not be taken lightly or overlooked in the morass of FMS symptoms. It has to be addressed equally with pain and fatigue.

Chronic hyperacidity of the stomach is another gastrointestinal problem. This condition causes an abnormal increase in production of stomach acid, which erodes the stomach lining and often contributes to the formation of peptic (stomach) or duodenal (intestinal) ulcers. The stomach and duodenum break down and digest foods using stomach acids and digestive enzymes. The duodenum is considered to be the first part of the small intestine located immediately beyond the stomach.

The second part of the small intestine is the jejunum, which absorbs nutrients from digested food. The third part of the small intestine is called the ileum and is where further absorption of food takes place. The ileum extends from the jejunum to a pouch-shape cecum, which connects it to the large intestine. Hyperacidity can cause several maladies, including peptic ulcer disease, where the hyperacidic stomach contributes to the formation of one or more chronic peptic ulcers on the stomach lining. Duodenal ulcers can also become a chronic problem.

Another condition, called gastritis, is a chronic inflammation of the mucous membrane that lines the stomach. This causes a break down in the integrity of areas in the stomach lining that shed, causing changes in gastric juices that leave the stomach vulnerable to bacterial attack and the formation of ulcers. This condition can be caused by the chronic over-stimulation of gastric juice production, such as pepsin, the primary enzyme produced in the stomach that breaks down proteins into simpler compounds for absorption in the small intestine.

Hyperacidity in the stomach is responsible for indigestion of all kinds, including esophageal burning. Hyperacidity can manifest as heartburn, abdominal pain and burning, bloating, excess gas, and general discomfort. Some sufferers find that Pepto-Bismol or a generic form of pink bismuth (made from a natural reddish-white crystalline metallic element) can be helpful. Although it does soothe an acidic stomach, this mixture is also used to sooth diarrhea and can slow down your bowels. If you are already suffering from constipation it can contribute to the problem. You may find that Alka Seltzer (containing a natural alkali mineral that dissolves gases) can soothe hyperacidity without worsening constipation. Sometimes the best remedy is plain old Tums, a calcium mineral antacid.

Be conservative when using these anti-acids. There are drugs that treat hyperacidity and all drugs come with side effects. Drinking the right amount of water each day can help dilute the excess acidity and wash it through your system. It is a good idea to stay away from strong spicy foods, chocolate, caffeine, alcohol, and acidic foods that can irritate the stomach lining and worsen hyperacidity. Like with all your other FMS symptoms, stress will make these conditions much worse, so protect yourself from stress.

5) Reproductive System and Urinary Tract

The reproductive system and urinary tract are home to some very unpleasant symptoms, especially for women, who make up the majority of FMS cases. The most predominant fibromyalgia symptom in the reproductive system is called vulvodynia, which is a complex condition including vulvitis (sore, even irritated to the point of being raw, vaginal lips), painful vaginal cramps or spasms with a burning discharge, increase in uterine menstrual cramps, and painful intercourse. These symptoms are not present in all female FMS patients, but when they occur it is important to see a gynecologist who is educated in fibromyalgia and who understands that these symptoms are part of your overall condition.

The most predominant fibromyalgia symptom in the urinary tract system is called chronic interstitial cystitis. This is a bladder condition that occurs predominantly in women and involves an inflammatory lesion or lesions located at the top of the bladder, which penetrate the entire thickness of the bladder wall. These lesions are called Hunner ulcers and are often difficult to detect because they can heal superficially; however, they are noted for their appearance as a small patch of brownish red mucosa surrounded by a network of radiating vessels. This condition can be accompanied by repeated bladder infections and concentrated, burning, and pungent urine. Again, if you have this symptom and seek the help of a specialist, make sure they know you have FMS and view interstitial cystitis as a symptom of a larger syndrome.

6) Dermis/Corium System (Skin)

The biological system called the dermis/corium refers to the "true skin" and includes a deep layer of skin called the epidermis, and a dense bed of vascular tissue. The dermis, or skin, is the organ that acts as our primary cooling system by releasing sweat, which is then cooled by the outside air. The skin also protects our body from invasion by bacteria and viruses. It is our outermost defense against the outside world.

The dermis is an organ with many parts, textures, thicknesses, and sensitivities. The skin consists of seven layers of dermal and sub-dermal cells which contain blood vessels, sweat and oil glands, skin pigmentation glands, and hair follicles that are in a constant state of production, self-replacement, and reaction to outside stimuli. When the outside temperature is cold the dermis shrinks up tight into "goose bumps," causing our body hair to stand up and insulate us from heat loss. In hot weather the dermis relaxes, opens up, and releases moisture to cool us down. The skin is really an amazing and busy organ, not to mention a crucial part of our overall state of health. Often the only part of our skin we take good care of is our face and the rest of it is uncared for until there is a problem.

When fibromyalgia manifests throughout the dermis it can be very miserable. Symptoms include: rashes in different sizes, shapes, thicknesses, and colors (red, pink or even brownish); bumps; raised areas; blotches; itching; burning; dullness; and soreness. With FMS, the dermis may feel as though it is burning all over, may radiate heat, may be itchy in unpredictable areas that do not exhibit a rash, and may produce a weird, "crawling" sensation, as though there are tiny worms moving just under the surface of the skin. Sometimes, the skin "buzzes" in areas that can be felt by another person. My husband said to me one night, "My God, you're buzzing!"

Sometimes the soles of the feet and/or the palms of the hands feel swollen, hot, itchy, or sweaty. There are also the "bee stings," which happen suddenly with no warning on the ankles, legs, or tips of the toes. Small, dry patches of pimples can appear on places like the back, outside of the upper arms, or the tops or backs of the thighs. The sweat glands can produce a kind of perspiration that is toxic and can irritate the skin. It is a good practice to drink enough water, take warm showers, not hot, and afterward use a gentle moisturizer all over the body, such as Cetaphil lotion or cream. For itching, take a warm bath in Epson Salts followed by gentle Cetaphil lotion or cream.

Using prescription creams that contain an anti-inflammatory, such as cortisone, can cause further problems. First of all, like with most drugs, the body develops a resistance to the strength of the original dose. Eventually, a higher strength is needed to offer the same relief as the original dose. Secondly, cortisone is a suppressant. When you suppress a symptom it goes deeper into the body, where it swelters and simmers. As soon as you discontinue the suppressant, the symptom can, and often does, return with a vengeance, like an angry seven-headed dragon suddenly awakened from its hibernation. Try to avoid this cycle if you can.

It is truly mind boggling how so many symptoms can fall under one umbrella and be a part of a single condition. The biggest mistake that a doctor can make is to misattribute FMS symptoms to another condition. With FMS, it is important to remember that each symptom is just that, a part of a larger illness; to look at each symptom as an individual problem will not help the healing process.

Chronic FMS is a paradox combining extreme dysenergism (inadequate energy/ATP production in the cells) along with the distortion and/or over-firing of bio-chemical impulses and signals to and from the brain. These impulses and signals travel from the brain into the body through the CNS along complex nerve pathways or "wires." So how is it possible to feel like you have absolutely no energy and also feel chronically overly stimulated at the same time? What causes the experience of the combined feelings of being completely and utterly exhausted together with a constant driving fight-or-flight anxiety (the feeling that something horrific or life-threatening is either happening or about to happen)? Chronic fibromyalgia is truly a mind-boggling paradox made in hell.

What on earth is going on here, and what is causing so many things to go haywire in the body all at once? Why does the body descend so far into energy deficit that it simply cannot generate enough energy to get itself out of debt, and falls into a serious energy bankruptcy? Is something affecting the body's energy production inside the cell matrixes? Is there some reason why the brain seems to have forgotten how to regulate and balance the bio-chemical electrical signals and impulses it sends throughout the body via central nervous system? Has the central nervous system blown a fuse?

It is important to note that the energy of the body (ATP) manufactured inside its cell matrixes is **not** the same thing as the bio-chemical nerve impulses that go to and from the brain meant to regulate the bodies biological systems and respond to outside stimuli. These are the two primary yet separate aspects of chronic fibromyalgia syndrome that affect the body, each in their particular ways. Aspect number one is a chronic energy deficit (dysenergism). Aspect number two is the distortion of brain signals and over-firing of the central nervous system. I will further explain this combined phenomenon in chapter thirteen under theories of physical causes. Be assured that although chronic fibromyalgia is **not** an easy condition to understand, it **can** be understood, made sense of and cured!

Freedom Light

Within the sorrow of what almost was
The visions in my soul are zephyrs that float through my being
like ghosts.
Ghosts of a time that was ripe with splendid joy; tragic, epic, and forever.
A time that endowed me with mystery.
A time that discovered me, and all I could ever be was revealed in one
transient eternity,
And brought forth, shared, and given with a force molten with
stern intent
To instill the essence of strength of being.
An inner strength that became unknown, unseen, or unfelt while living a
Thrown upon life, only to be revealed in one timely instant,
To emerge like an awakened dragon from its restorative cave,
To leave the darkness and spread its sleepy wings without,
To expose the giant and hidden heart within.
A heart that has fought so bravely,
A heart always so steadfast, so heavy, and so carried among and through
The irreverent course, and around the bends of unfriendly miles
That wound sharply into hazes and disappeared.
A heart yet carried forth to dare the journey to hold itself
Against a truer and more sublimely intended fate.
A fate to find its freedom light, to illuminate each struggle,
And to see that the strength, the courage, and the love intended
Was only moments away, and always present within, to be sought out
Through this determined agony, and claimed forever as rightful.
To be melded together with every gift so freely given, as this giant and
Brave heart begins to pass through each new and given day.

Valerie Lumley

Chapter Five
Theories of Psychological Causes

On November 10, 1493, in Einsiedeln, Switzerland, the only son of a poor German physician of noble decent was born. Christened Theophrastus Bombastus von Hohenheim, he later renamed himself Philippus Aureolus Paracelsus and became known simply as Paracelsus. Around 1510, Paracelsus received his bachelor's degree in chemistry and medicine at the University of Basel, and soon afterward earned a doctorate degree and studied under the Hermetic philosopher, Trithemius.

Between 1510 and 1524, Paracelsus wandered through Europe, Russia, and the Middle East as a military surgeon, an experience which provided him with considerable amount of knowledge in alchemy. During his travels he became acquainted with remedies unfamiliar to the contemporary physicians of his time, which brought him notably high prestige.

Paracelsus set out to reform medicine by opposing the ways of scholastic physicians and medical authorities and emphasizing the importance of practical knowledge. When he was accused of using poisons (non-organic as well as organic internal remedies), he introduced the idea that his opponents used "poisons" when they prescribed improper dosages of their medicines. After introducing the idea of dosages, he introduced the idea of experimentation to find the right medicine for the right malady. Paracelsus was also noted for teaching the revolutionary idea that wounds would heal naturally when kept clean and drained.

In 1526, Paracelsus became professor of medicine at the University of Basel. He boldly and publicly burned the guiding works of his predecessors, proclaiming that his "cap had in it more learning than all the heads in the university." During this time, Paracelsus continued to write prolifically about the ancient Hermetic system of medicine. In 1528, Paracelsus was driven out of Basel after a quarrel with the magistracy. After wandering in Switzerland and southern Germany, he settled for a few years in the Province of Carinthia in Austria, where he produced some of his most famous writings. It is believed Paracelsus was poisoned or killed by assassins hired by his enemies. He died in Salzburg on September 23, 1541.

Despite the criticism Paracelsus received for his obsession with alchemy, he encouraged research and observation. He improved pharmacy and therapeutics and revolutionized the medical methods of his time through his extensive experimentation. He was among the first to write scientific books for public use and, in 1589, a complete edition of his works was released for the first time in Latin. Paracelsus' writings used the esoteric terminology of the Rosicrucian scholars of his time, i.e. the language of the Brotherhood of the Rosy Cross.

This language used expressions that were alive, terse, and denoted "complexes," or meanings derived from the esoterically empirical knowledge of the Rosicrucian. Because the language was so specialized, a problem of interpretation arose; words often meant something entirely different in this vocabulary than they did in the vernacular of the times. Even highly intelligent scholars, if not trained in this language, would have mistaken much of Paracelsus' meaning.

Based on the Hermetic principle of interrelationship, Paracelsus was the first physician to recognize the connection between the human psyche and the physical organism, thus paving the way for the future work of Mesmer and, subsequently, Freud. Paracelsus was known for his mixed bag of beliefs and, due to the abnormal nature of his work, was looked upon unfavorably. However, Paracelsus later became known as the Pathfinder, the Innovator whose fame as the founder of a new school of medicine earned him a title as "one of the fathers of modern medicine."

The character of Paracelsus has inspired the works of many writers, among them Carl Jung, whose "Psychology and Alchemy," written in 1944, was heavily influenced by Paracelsus' work. In his book "The Occult Causes of Disease," author E. Wolfram writes a compendium of the teachings of Paracelsus' "Volumen Paramirum." Wolfram's book contains the words of Paracelsus, translated as accurately as possible, considering the difficult nature of its language. The word "occult," in this context, means something beyond human understanding, mysterious, secret, covered, not divulged or disclosed, hidden, veiled, or concealed from view.

A quote from Paracelsus in Wolfram's book refers to theories of causes where Paracelsus states the cause of all disease is occult. He said, "It is the fate of the Art of Healing in our time that it has had to rely upon theories; theories which are the deduction drawn from effects which have become manifest; manifestations which in their turn again are the result of occult activities. It is also the fate of our times that its knowledge is largely drawn from the realm of hypothesis, and that in consequence, hypothetical statements and knowledge become mistaken one for the other - with the result that what 'alone' is true to-day, runs that chance of having practically 'no value' in ten years time. And what here holds good for the ills of the body holds good also for the ills affecting the soul."

Paracelsus saw that today's medicine became out-dated tomorrow, but he also believed that the weakening of the soul leaves the body vulnerable to disease. He insisted that there is a connection between the state of a person's soul, their physical health, and the nature of the Art of Healing prevalent at any given time. He also believed in what he called the real meaning of the word "physiology," which he defined as "the study of the nature of the soul." Paracelsus accepted the soul as reality, rather than as a convenient hypothesis. I believe that understanding this relationship between body and soul is crucial to the healing process.

The foresight of Paracelsus is astonishingly ahead of his time; he has revealed the pitfalls of using theory and hypothesis in diagnosis, he has referenced predispositions to certain conditions, he has suggested that life stressors can trigger these predispositions, and he has found great insight concerning the connection between the soul and the body.

Paracelsus' writings repeatedly imply the belief that only experience can create knowledge, therefore a theory or a hypothesis is not equivalent to knowing something, nor should it be considered fact. This precedes Albert Einstein's famous quote, "True knowledge can only come from experience." Even with the cloud of skepticism that seemed to hover over Paracelsus throughout his career, his perceptions and conclusions still provide sound guidance in today's modern world of medical treatment. Paracelsus was considered one of the few mystics of his time who committed to "scale those heights which had hitherto seemed beyond man's reach, and it became the Path upon which many a one filled with devotion now set his feet, but few dared to pursue to its loftiest summit." It was from the knowledge of these few that the origin of disease was set down by Paracelsus under the disguise of carefully veiled occult terminology.

Paracelsus noted the cause of all disease quoted as:
- The influence of climate and infection.
- Poisons, such as man's organism compels him to take up in the process of eating, drinking, and breathing, as well as through the medium of his organs of perception.
- The manner in which the body was conditioned at birth.
- Magic and Spiritual influences.
- God's will, or "karma."

These occult wisdoms from the different Schools of Intuition before Paracelsus' time pertaining to the Devine Gift of Healing were reflected in the works of the sages (the early philosophers). It may be beneficial to bear in mind the ancient wisdom and knowledge when considering the theories of today.

There are many theories regarding the cause of chronic FMS and it is worth it to view them with an open yet skeptical mind, and to do so honestly. A simple and well-known theory is that fibromyalgia is caused by a combination of stress, trauma, and environmental toxins. The Chinese call fibromyalgia "wind in the body," meaning a virus that has taken up residence and cannot be evicted by a weakened immune system.

In 2008, The World Gene Congress in China reported that 90% of all cells in the body are active bacterial cells and only 10% are human. They also stated that there is an imbalance of approximately 1,000,000 bacterial genes to only 25,000 human genes in the body. At this Congress, Dr. Trevor Marshall indicated that chronic diseases, such as Chronic Fatigue Syndrome, and autoimmune diseases, such as Lupus, could be attributed to this imbalance.

Many of these theories involve both psychological and physical causes. The Paracelsian model for the origin of disease is an interesting model, although it does not include factors such as physical injury and synthetic medications.

Theories of Psychological Causes

In 1875, the effects of the mind on the body were comprehensively assigned by an enlightened woman named Mary Baker Eddie (1821-1908), who published her work in a volume called "Science and Health With Key to the Scriptures." In 1879, Mrs. Eddie was responsible for forming "The First Church of Christ, Scientist," which holds today. Some basic principles, or spiritual truths, that form the foundation of this faith are simple: "There is no life, truth or intelligence in matter. All is infinite mind and its infinite manifestation." Other beliefs held by this faith are: thoughts externalize themselves; illness is a manifestation of wrong thinking (error); and right thinking is capable of healing. While I will not argue with the fact that negative thought patterns have the ability to affect us physically, there are times when the human body acts outside of its mental influence.

I will venture to say that even though I believe the spirit is perfect, I also recognize that the body is material—it is not indestructible, nor is it infallible. Just because an unhealthy state of mind can cause illness does not mean all illness is caused by an unhealthy state of mind. Illness can be caused when a physical error occurs on its own, such as a triggered genetic predisposition, or when external forces act upon the body such as an accidental injury or an invading microorganism.

Today, medical specialists tend to look only where previous experience has led them; doctors often only analyze symptoms which fall into their field. This may complicate straightforward symptoms and make them appear to be more important than they are; even while looking through the highly polished lens of a medical specialty, sometimes a cigar is just a cigar, and the simplicity of this dynamic can evade some doctors. Before considering various psychological theories as possible causes for chronic FMS, remember that the science of psychology is a relatively new one.

Look how far the science of psychology has evolved since the Freudian era. The scientific methods of today are not infallible and data can easily be misinterpreted. For this reason, when researching possible psychological causes for FMS, use your common sense and personal experiences to determine whether a theory is probable or not in relation to you. What you know through personal experience can serve as an invaluable barometer.

Somatoform Disorders

Cited from the DSM (diagnostic statistical manual for mental illnesses), a somatoform disorder is "the presence of physical symptoms that suggest a general medical condition." These symptoms must feature significant distress or impairment in occupational and social functionality and must be involuntary.

Psychological disorders dealing with physical pain and chronic illness that fall under the category of Somatoform Disorders are: Somatization Disorder; Undifferentiated Somatoform Disorder; Conversion Disorder; Pain Disorder; and Hypochondriasis. Hypochondriasis, Conversion Disorder, and Pain Disorder are the most feasible hypothetical causes of FMS in this category, so we will further investigate them.

1) Hypochondriasis (Diagnostic code #300.7)
Diagnostic criteria for Hypochondriasis, according to the DSM

- An occupation with fears of having, or the idea that one has, a serious disease based on the person's misinterpretation of bodily symptoms.
- This preoccupation persists despite appropriate medical evaluation and reassurance.

- The belief in Criterion A is not of delusional intensity and is not restricted to a circumscribed concern about appearance.
- The preoccupation causes clinically significant distress or impairment in social, occupational or other important areas of functioning.
- The duration of the disturbance is at least 6 months.
- The preoccupation is not better accounted for by another form of Somatoform Disorder.

Criterion B says that Hypochondriasis is present if symptoms are not proven by testing. The problem here lies in the fact that there are no known clinical tests to confirm the presence of FMS, and this fact alone does not mean that FMS is a manifestation of Hypochondriasis.

Under criterion C the patient is capable of acknowledging the possibility that he or she may be exaggerating a feared disease and can admit there may be no disease at all. If, during a current episode, a patient is not able to recognize the possibility that their concern may be excessive or unreasonable (although it never becomes delusional), then the specified "with poor insight" is used with the diagnosis.

There are also other associated features to this mental disorder:
- A lengthy history is often presented in great detail.
- The patient engages in "doctor shopping."
- There is often anger and frustration in the doctor/patient relationships on both sides and the patient often believes he or she is not getting the proper care.
- The patient may resist referral to a mental health professional.
- The patient repeatedly initiates risky diagnostic procedures that can be costly and can sometimes cause complications to arise.
- The patient can experience intrusive thoughts about a disease with associated compulsive behavior.

This behavior is likely to receive only a cursory evaluation, which is often not thorough enough to detect an underlying condition. The stress of coping with Hypochondriasis may spill over into other areas of the patient's life by causing strained social and professional relationships, and may become completely disabling.

Hypochondriasis is a chronic condition that is often accompanied by other mental disorders. Because of the chronic nature of this condition the most important factor in considering this diagnosis lies in looking for a differential diagnosis, or the existence of an underlying general medical condition.

If the patient manifests early stages of an endocrine condition (such as thyroid or parathyroid disease), a neurological condition (such as multiple sclerosis or myasthenia gravis), diseases that affect multiple body systems (such as lupus erythematosus or fibromyalgia), or occult malignancies, then the condition of Hypochondriasis may not be a factor.

The DSM generally states that, although Hypochondriasis can itself be a co-existing condition, if there is an acute onset of symptoms, an absence of a Personality Disorder, and an absence of a "secondary gain" (being relieved of responsibilities, getting more attention and so on) then Hypochondriasis is not the correct diagnosis. This was my conclusion in examining my own case.

To help in my healing process, my therapist recommended that I take a personality test. When I got the results back, they did not describe who I thought I was at all. The test had determined that, while I was a "sincere and likeable person," I was also a hysterical hypochondriac who plagued my relationships with emotional problems. The test results also reported that these emotional problems were not real, but were manifestations of my unconscious hysteria. Finding this odd, I tried to talk to my therapist about the results. She assured me that the test I took was a "standardized test" and was considered to be reliable and accurate.

Beyond perplexed, I tried to explain the discrepancy between what the test results revealed and who I really was. My therapist explained that my implied hysteria was on the subconscious level, so I naturally was unaware of it. I tried to tell her that anyone who knew me would dismiss this test immediately, as my husband had done, but she would not concede that the test could be wrong.

I have become more aware of my body since the onset of FMS, and I will admit that I have, on a few occasions, reacted to my symptoms in a hysterical way; however, this increase in awareness and hysterical behavior began after FMS had set in, not before. I believe that my reactions to the many different kinds of pain I have experienced are typical of anyone who has gone through a similar illness. Anyone who deals with intense pain for years would get hysterical at some point.

Practically speaking, I tend to reject the premise that unconscious impulses are wholly unknown to the conscious mind, even though the unconscious is sometimes said to be a guiding force behind our conscious choices. It has been my experience that messages from the unconscious mind can be observed by the conscious mind and vise versa. For example, unfounded, unconscious fears and anxieties can not only be observed, they can be negated by consciously feeding the inner mind messages that are informed, appropriate, and rational. By feeding your subconscious educated facts about whatever it is you are afraid of you can reverse the fear, even if you feel you have no control over it.

Through my experiences, I have chosen to dismiss Hypochondriasis as a possible cause of FMS. I know that I am not a hysterical hypochondriac, so I know that this is not the cause of my illness; however, I am now aware that hysteria can occur and, because it causes stress that could exacerbate FMS, I use this new knowledge to avoid hysterical episodes which would worsen my condition and I focus on remaining calm.

This link between the mind and the body, between stress and physical pain, is crucial. I took the two and a half hour personality test at a time when I was in severe pain and had to sit up at a desk that was too high and in a chair that was too low. Several times I had to lie down on the floor on pillows I took from the chairs in the waiting room, to try to relieve the severe pain in my shoulders and neck.

The following day I went to see my Osteopath for osteopathic manipulation therapy to relieve the pain in my back, neck, and shoulders. He said I was such a mess he had to give me a trio of a muscle relaxer, an anti-inflammatory, and a pain reliever to take for two weeks before he would attempt to treat me. He was angry at the conditions under which I was expected to take the test and very concerned about my physical state.

If I knew at the time how potentially vulnerable I was to the consequences of taking this kind of psychological test, I would not have so eagerly volunteered to take it. Unaware that the test would damage my progress, I took it in the hope of acquiring some useful information that might be helpful to my healing.

If your doctor is convinced that your symptoms are due to Hyperchondriasis, do not feel bad about finding a new physician. You are the only one who knows the intensity of your pain, and you need a doctor who believes in the severity of your symptoms; otherwise, you will not receive the medical care you need and deserve. Until a deeper understanding of chronic FMS is attainable you will have to forge your own path through its labyrinth of stigmas and misdiagnoses.

2) Conversion Disorder (Diagnostic code #300.11)
Diagnostic criteria for Conversion Disorder according to the DSM are as follows:

- One or more symptoms or deficits affecting voluntary motor or sensory functions that suggest a neurological or other general medical condition.
- Psychological factors are judged to be associated with the symptom or deficit because the initiation or exacerbation of the symptom or deficit is preceded by psychological stressors.
- The symptom or deficit is not intentionally produced or feigned (as in Factitious Disorder or Malingering).

- The symptom or deficit cannot be fully explained by a general medical condition or by the direct effects of a substance, or as a culturally sanctioned behavior or experience.
- The symptom or deficit causes clinically significant distress or impairment in social, occupational, or other important areas of functioning, or warrants medical evaluation.
- The symptom or deficit is not limited to pain or sexual dysfunction and does not occur exclusively during the course of Somatization Disorder or another mental disorder.

The DSM generally states that Conversion Disorder symptoms are typically called pseudo neurological because they are related to voluntary sensory or motor function. Voluntary sensory symptoms include: double vision; blindness; deafness; loss of touch or pain sensation; hallucinations; and may also include convulsions and seizures. Voluntary motor symptoms include: impaired coordination or balance; localized weakness or paralysis; difficulty swallowing with a sensation of a lump in the throat; and urinary retention.

Due to these confusing and complex symptoms, a broad range of neurological conditions may be misdiagnosed as Conversion Disorder, so it is very important that a thorough medical investigation is performed to rule out other general conditions. Also, since the manifestation of certain conditions may take years before they become evident, and due to the fact that as many as one third of patients with conversion symptoms have a current or prior neurological condition (including FMS), a diagnosis of Conversion Disorder should only be viewed as tentative or provisional when it is made.

Conversion Disorder can be ruled out as a theory of cause for chronic FMS for a number of reasons. First, the onset of Conversion Disorder is generally after age ten and before age 35, while FMS can onset at any age. Second, if Conversion Disorder does develop during mid to old age the probability is high that the patient has an occult neurological condition or another general medical condition.

Third, conversion symptoms come on very quickly and acutely, and are not chronic, like the symptoms of FMS. Although conversion symptoms can recur, this happens only in one fifth to one quarter of patients within the first year only, whereas the great majority of FMS patients experience the misery of recurrent or chronic symptoms year after year.

Fourth, the only factors that are associated with a favorable prognosis in Conversion Disorder are the presence of a clearly identifiable stress at the time of its onset, immediate treatment, and in a patient with above average intelligence. These criteria do not include a physical trauma or injury as a triggering factor, as it is in the case of most chronic FMS onsets. In addition, neither immediate treatment nor the patient's intelligence are proven as contributing factors in the success of reversing chronic FMS.

3) Pain Disorders (Diagnostic code #307.80 and #307.89)
Diagnostic criteria for Pain Disorders according to the DMS are as follows:

- Pain in one or more anatomical sites is the predominant focus of the clinical presentation, and is of sufficient severity to warrant clinical attention.
- The pain causes clinically significant distress or impairment in social, occupational, or other important areas of functioning.
- Psychological factors are judged to have an important role in the onset, severity, exacerbation, or maintenance of the pain.
- The symptoms are not intentionally produced or feigned (as in Factitious Disorder or Malingering).
- The pain is not better accounted for by a mood, anxiety, or psychotic disorder and does not meet the criteria for Dyspareunia (pain during sexual intercourse).

Pain Disorders are defined by diagnostic codes #307.80 and #307.89. Diagnostic code #307.80 is distinguished if psychological factors are judged to be crucial in the onset, severity, exacerbation, or maintenance of the pain, and if a general medical condition does not play a major role.

Diagnostic code # 307.89 is distinguished if both psychological factors and a general medical condition are judged to have important roles in the onset, severity, exacerbation, or maintenance of the pain. This pain disorder typically reveals some kind of pathology associated with the pain or a general medical condition, such as various musculoskeletal conditions. These include a wide variety of conditions such as disc herniation, osteoporosis, rheumatoid arthritis, and myofascial pain syndrome.

Also included in this list are neuropathies, such as diabetic neuropathy, post-herpetic neuralgia, and occult malignancies, such as metastatic lesions in the bone or tumorous infiltration of some nerves. A common denominator among this variety of conditions is that any attempt to treat the pain often causes the level of pain to increase. The DSM does not yet mention chronic fibromyalgia syndrome as a possible general medical condition associated with pain, however I believe it should be added.

There are several associated features of Pain Disorder that can be summed up in general terms. In spite of the fact that there is a wide range of variability in the onset of chronic pain, it seems that in this disorder chronic pain appears to be most frequently associated with Depressive Disorders. It is well known that depression can cause a downward spiral in overall health. This spiral begins with a painful psychological problem that causes the depression. The depression then manifests into the body as pain, which causes social isolation that leads to more psychological problems and depression, causing even more pain.

This result is a reduction of physical activity that causes physical endurance to decline, fatigue to set in, and more pain to occur. Pain Disorders may occur at any age, appear more in females than in males, and cause chronic back pain, which disables ten to fifteen percent of known adult cases in the United States. In most cases, the pain symptoms persist for several years prior to the patient being referred to a mental health professional.

After acknowledging that chronic depression can manifest as pain, it is important to remember:

- Chronic FMS is triggered in most cases by a compounding minor or major injury, or physical trauma.
- Nearly all FMS patients experience chronic depression as a natural byproduct of the condition.
- The stress of this subsequent depression exacerbates FMS symptoms.
- Stress exacerbates the symptoms of any illness or condition.

For these reasons, I do not believe that Pain Disorder can be realistically considered a cause of chronic FMS. Even though chronic FMS can be accompanied by a psychological disorder, not everyone with FMS has a psychological disorder and not everyone with a psychological disorder has FMS. Therefore, a causal link between the two factors cannot be made.

Only you and your health care providers can decide if a somatoform component accompanies your FMS. If any of the above criteria seems to describe your condition, look into it as a possible symptom of your illness. Be honest with yourself; FMS is a difficult disease to diagnose, so do not settle for the wrong diagnosis in the hopes that your medical struggles will end.

I believe that when you have chronic FMS, a reversible form of pain syndrome can eventually become a part of the illness. Stress and depression can add to the downward spiral of pain and weakness in FMS, making it difficult to determine what is actually causing the pain. Everyday we face stress, both psychological and physical, and it is important for you, as an FMS sufferer, to be able to tell the difference between the stressors of FMS itself, the normal everyday stressors, and those severe enough to exacerbate your condition.

Effects of Stress on the Body

Stress is one of modern society's biggest monsters. If this monster is in your life, it must be contained and managed, never allowed to run amuck, and eliminated whenever possible. The term stress, which is one of the most frequently used words in our society, is generally used in reference to a mental, emotional, or physical strain. It also refers to any reaction to a mental, emotional, physical, or social stimulus requiring a response that is different from the way we normally think, feel, or react.

Bad stress (distress) can come from many sources, such as suppressed negative emotions like frustration, hate, rage, anxiety, fear, or grief, or from on-going intense relationship problems. It can also come from being chronically over-worked, put under too much physical or psychological pressure, or living with a severe, chronic illness. Bad stress can be extremely detrimental to overall physical and mental health and seriously exacerbates fibromyalgia symptoms.

Good stress (eustress) comes from things like excitement, joy, elation, exhilaration, sex, or pleasurable physical activities, such as exercise or sports. Good stress is temporary and a normal, healthy part of life; it poses no health problems because it only causes a short-term release of norephinephrine, which helps to create new memories, improves mood, and stimulates creative thought, which encourages the brain to create more synaptic connections. However, for a fibromyalgic, even good stress can cause a painful flare-up because any sudden draw on the body's energy puts a strain on an already overdrawn system.

It is almost as though someone with severe FMS is not allowed to feel the stress of any high-level emotions. When people turn to comfort food, alcohol, or cigarettes to relieve or control stress they cause more stress for their bodies.

Stress can damage the brain. An article written by the Institute for Natural Resources (INR) in 2006 reports that clinical studies show increased levels of cortisol can damage and even shrink the gray matter of the brain, particularly the limbic system, which is associated with basic needs, and the hippocampus, which is responsible for learning and memory. This happens because the limbic system and the hippocampus are not the part of the brain involved in the stress response. In the case of long-term stress, these areas of the brain undergo atrophy because they are not being activated enough, and become increasing sensitivity to stress hormone cortisol. This means that the areas of the brain that are involved in the stress response are over-stimulated, to the detriment of the areas that are not involved.

These studies also reveal evidence that stress accelerates the aging of the brain. When chronic stress continually bathes the brain in stress hormones intended for a short-term emergency response, it causes the brain to actually shrink and produce abnormal glial cell function. Glial cells, which nourish nerve cells in the brain and spinal cord, along with neurons, make up the majority of brain cells. When chronic stress persists, these brain cells are damaged and eventually die. The result is an increased rate of "wear and tear" on the brain regions frequently activated during stress. Researchers estimate that stress is a major exacerbation to 80% of all major illnesses and is also a common precursor to the development of psychological problems, such as depression and anxiety. Although stress is generally viewed as a psychological problem, its physical effects are very real.

Like clinical depression, which sends painful biochemical shock waves through the body, ordinary stress is harmful to the mind and the body. The mental ramifications of stress include: panic attacks; anxiety; obsessive-compulsive disorder; post-traumatic stress disorder; dissociative disorder; and other phobic disorders. Physical ramifications of stress include a variety of digestive disorders, such as peptic ulcer disease and irritable bowel syndrome. Distress comes in two basic forms, each with its own biochemistry.

Acute Stress

The first form of stress is acute stress, which is an immediate response to imminent danger. This response floods the body with a surge of powerful stress hormones that can have a very damaging effect on the cardiovascular system. This is the primal "fight or flight" response that was once crucial for the survival of our ancestors and is still laced within our DNA as an automatic response to sudden stimulation, whether it be life threatening or not.

The fight or flight response begins in the hypothalamus, the amygdala, which is associated with fear and aggression, and the pituitary gland, which controls glands associated with metabolism. These three structures exchange information with and send hormones and nerve signals to the rest of the body; these signals are meant to prepare the body to immediately respond to the unexpected stimulus.

The adrenal glands dump heavy amounts of adrenaline, also called epinephrine, into the bloodstream, causing the heart to beat faster, the blood pressure to increase, and the lungs to work harder to fill the body with oxygen. The pituitary gland increases its production of adrenocorticotropic hormones (ACTH), which stimulate the adrenal medulla. The adrenal medulla releases high levels of cortisol, cortisone, and other glucocorticoids into the bloodstream to help the body convert its stores of sugar and fat into fast accessible energy. As a result, cholesterol levels rise and the blood composition changes, making it more prone to clotting, which increases the likelihood of a stroke or a heart attack.

The adrenals also release a heavy amount of adrenaline and norepinephrine, which act as the principle neurotransmitters for the sympathetic nerve endings that supply signals to the major organs, muscles, and skin. This causes the muscles to tense and the senses to sharpen in preparation for a fast action response. The last thing to happen in this stunning biochemical cascade is the slowing and eventual shut down of digestion.

After the threat passes, the acute responses turn off and the production of stress hormones ceases, allowing the body to relax. If the fight or flight response is initiated too often serious damage can be done to the body, especially the arterial walls. In today's society it is near impossible to get away from stress and, although not all the distress we encounter is due to physical threats, the body's reaction is the same.

Chronic Stress

The second form of stress, called chronic or long-term stress, occurs when a person is constantly exposed to emotional or psychological pressures he or she cannot always control. This pressure can come from any source, such as an abusive and/or dysfunctional relationship with a close family member, spouse, friend or an employer that has unreasonable expectations. Chronic stress is particularly dangerous because it eventually wears the body out. Because of the way it weakens the immune system, long-term stress causes the body to be more susceptible to illness and slows down healing.

Persistent stress causes the body to maintain a near constant circulation of the glucocorticoids cortisol, cortisone, and adrenaline, which are collectively referred to as the stress hormones and are produced in the adrenal gland. Prolonged exposure can lead to many complications, including: chronic tension in the muscles; a weakened immune system; the destruction of T-cells; the loss of bone mass; the suppression of the reproductive system; and memory problems. T-cells, in particular, are a critical part of the body's defense against disease; without T-cells the body will be extremely vulnerable to cancer and infection. Research has shown that patients with chronic fibromyalgia are 35% more at risk of developing cancer, due to severely weakened immune systems and the subsequent destruction of vital T-cells.

The adverse effects to the body's overall health caused by chronic, long-term stress can be quite serious. The adrenal gland's production of stress hormones is said to be responsible for the majority of symptoms and ailments associated with stress. At the top of the list of these symptoms are nutritional deficiencies. When the adrenals increase their production of adrenaline, the body speeds up the metabolism of proteins, fats, and carbohydrates to produce fast energy for the body. This in turn causes the body to excrete amino acids, potassium, and phosphorus, to deplete its stores of magnesium in muscle tissue, and to store less calcium, which results in loss of bone mass.

Because chronic stress slows digestion, the body cannot readily break down and absorb ingested nutrients. This causes deficiencies in: B-complex vitamins, which contribute to the healthy functioning of the nervous system; electrolytes; and the promotion of free radical formations, which cause damage to cell membranes and body tissues and are often associated with stress.

Identifying The Source of Your Stress

Identifying and acknowledging the sources of your stress will help you begin to find ways to contain it and manage it whenever possible, and eliminate it whenever necessary. In *Prescriptions for Natural Healing* there is a classic list of stressors, which begins with the most severe:

- Death of a child, spouse, or other close family member
- Divorce
- Death of a close friend
- Financial problems
- Legal separation from spouse
- Job loss
- Major injury
- New marriage
- Scheduled surgery
- Change in family member's health
- Serious trouble at work
- Increased responsibility at work or home
- Sexual problems
- Change of jobs
- Child leaving home
- Change in residence
- Major change in diet
- Vacation
- Allergies

I find it interesting to see that a widely accepted stress list does not include chronic illness or sudden and complete disability. From my experience, the loss of your way of life to a chronic illness is extremely stressful, and I would personally rank it near the top of this list.

Chronic FMS is a major, life altering, and terrifying condition that continuously stresses the body and the mind. This illness creates a degree of stress that cannot be ignored. Although you cannot completely rid your life of stress, there is a lot you can do to create a low-stress environment. Learning to contain, manage, and balance the mental and emotional stress that is absolutely unavoidable for daily living is a good place to start, especially if you are living with chronic FMS. You may need to leave a job, a city, a spouse, a biological family member, or a friend, but health benefits provided by the stress reduction will be worth it.

If you do not need to make a major life change in order to control your stress level, instead, try to: employ frequent time outs and rests; learn to pick your battles; avoid unnecessary hassles; change a stressful routine; set healthy boundaries; remember to laugh and enjoy life; pursue a hobby; practice relaxation, meditation, and deep breathing techniques; and do not let your emotions build up, allow them expression and be honest with yourself about why you feel how you do.

It is your responsibility to manage your mental and emotional stress, remove any excess stress in your life, and make a conscious effort to make monitoring your stress a part of your daily routine.

Three Ways to Combat Stress

Sufficient Sleep: The primary physical and nutritional consequences of stress can also be managed, balanced, and reversed. The most important thing you can do for your physical body is to get regular, sufficient sleep, so that your body is not deprived of the chance to repair itself from the ravages of the day. If you find you cannot sleep, you can use a mild sleep aid. Make sure, though, that you use the lowest dose possible and do not make it a habit.

Nutritional Considerations: The next most important thing you can do for the body is to pay attention to nutritional considerations. You can begin by eating a diet that helps the body produce ATP (cellular energy). Eating 50% to 75% of your daily diet of fresh, raw, and dark colored fruits and vegetables is a good place to start. These foods will not only supply the body with valuable vitamins and minerals, they are rich in vitamin-C compounds called bioflavonoids, which come from the pigmentation found in the pectin of many dark colored fruits and plants.

These bioflavonoids are called anti-oxidants because they scavenge and neutralize the damage caused by dangerous free radicals, which are single oxygen molecules responsible for breaking down and destroying cells. Avoid foods that quickly and easily convert into fast energy, such as processed foods. These foods are typically white foods such as sugar, white flour, pasta, potatoes, and white rice.

Also, limit red meat, eggs, pork, fried food, fast food, foods containing preservatives, carbonated sodas, and unnatural artificial sweeteners, such as aspartame. A good friend of mine who has FMS told me she felt much better when she eliminated carbonated drinks all together. Eating very small quantities of dark chocolate can be a mood elevator; however, milk chocolate should be avoided because of its high sugar and high fat content. Dairy products can contribute to a "nervous" condition in some people, so you can try eliminating them for three weeks and then bring them back slowly while monitoring their effects.

Limiting your intake of caffeine is very important because it makes you nervous and disrupts normal sleep patterns, like sugar does. Also avoid alcohol because it is a neurotoxin and aggravates nerve pain. Smoking cigarettes is also a toxic habit that should be broken.

Gentle Physical Exercise: Finally, getting some form of regular gentle physical exercise every day, if possible, has proven indispensable for FMS patients. I realize how painful it can be for a fibromyalgia patient to move around, and the severe pain of FMS makes it very difficult for its sufferers to begin and sustain a regular exercise program. Any kind of exertion on the muscles can flare-up nerve and muscle pain temporarily, however increasing flexibility in the muscles will reduce pain and stress, prevent the body from deteriorating into a state of muscular atrophy, and help prevent the downward spiral caused by overall physical weakness.

Once you become completely deconditioned with atrophied muscles, it can take up to a year or more to get your strength back. A physical therapist told me that researchers have found that it can take up to 22,000 movements over time for a single muscle to regain its tone and strength after it has deteriorated into a state of atrophy. Once you are in an overall weakened state the cycle of pain continues, as weakness contributes to fatigue, which causes more pain, which contributes to more weakness, etc. Gentle physical exercise is the only way to prevent this cycle from taking complete control of your life.

Try walking short distances at regular intervals a few times a day. Walking is a weight bearing exercise that gets the entire body moving and the blood flowing. A few gentle stretches can also be good. Never use weights with any form of exercise. If stretching on a hard or padded floor is too painful, try doing some stretches with the support of your bed. Do what feels least painful and most natural. If walking or stretching is too painful, or you are too weak to exercise on land against the earth's gravitational pull, then try a warm-water pool physical therapy program. The water will support your weight and the warmth will sooth the pain and relax your muscles while you get them moving.

Talk to your doctor to get a prescription for a warm-water pool exercise program in your area (about 93 degrees). Start somewhere, keep going, and be very patient. It will get easier, your body will begin to feel better, and your mind will become clearer. If you can begin with doing some slow and gentle Tai Chi, you can gradually move up to gentle restorative Yoga or a gentle, modified form of Pilates. Personally, I find restorative yoga to be the most affective way to lengthen and strengthen muscles and balance the body. Regular gentle physical exercise will help reduce the pain and stress in your life, increase flexibility and strength, improve balance and mental clarity, and can even reduce blood pressure.

As for the theory that stress can be the sole cause of chronic fibromyalgia syndrome, you can see that it can certainly make it worse in many ways. However I do not see how the effects of stress can fully account for the vast, mixed bag of symptoms that are so characteristic of FMS. While I strongly believe that stress exacerbates FMS and can block any chance of healing it completely, I also believe that there is an occult underlying physical component to the cause of chronic FMS.

Although research has shown that stress from a minor physical or psychological trauma has played a major role in triggering a substantial amount of full-blown chronic FMS cases, I believe that, even in these cases, an underlying physical component exists.

Depression

Like a thick blanket of dense fog, depression silently engulfs your entire world, covering everything that had formerly been clearly visible and known to you as real. This relentless, unstoppable force overtakes you without mercy. It infiltrates your body and your mind like a calculating, well-trained enemy spy on a silent mission to sabotage and destroy all hope. You feel yourself being compressed downward into a terrifying and foreign world beneath the surface of your former perceptions, where everything seems vague and unreal like a hazy non-existence.

Depression can make you feel as if the ground is sinking beneath you and each effort to gain a foothold is a struggle. As you sink further and further into a soggy quagmire of confusion and uncertainty, the memory of your former world begins to fade. Your life-force seems to drain away in every direction, your senses begin to dull, your mind begins to float off into the distance, and your spirit begins to sink deep into a murky pool. Your entire being seems to simultaneously disperse into nothingness.

The fog of depression covers your home, it seeps in through every window and door and fills every room, corner, cabinet and drawer. It permeates your clothes, runs out the faucets and floats out the heating ducts, filling the air. It coats the walls, floor, furniture and ceiling. Depression is everywhere causing pain in every way. It shuts you down and snuffs you out, and in doing so it affects you, everyone and everything around you that was once a vital part of your life. It steals away the life you once knew and the person you once were and it does so without your consent, without your intension, and without warning.

Depression blurs the lines separating reality and unreality, causing them to gradually seem to become one and soon the confusion and uncertainty from the continuous presence of this melded dichotomy begins to make you feel crazy. As depression takes over your life, your body and your mind, the inner voices begin to softly chant in low tones the incoherent insinuations of worthlessness and self-loathing. As you lose your appetite and ability to sleep undisturbed, your energy and thoughts sink even lower and the future seems bleak, pointless and unreachable.

The effects of depression, such as loss of appetite, the inability to sleep, thoughts of suicide, and loss of energy, can make any attempt to regain your previous state of health pointless. Don't let the hopelessness of depression take control; depression can occur for any number of reasons, but it does not have to ruin your life.

Causes of Depression

There are many causes for depression. A 2003 article in a special edition of Time Magazine, entitled *"How Your Mind Can Heal Your Body,"* states that more and more patients and doctors are realizing that physical and mental wellbeing are inseparable. It is now acknowledged that an unhealthy mind can lead to an unhealthy body by triggering a physical illness or by exacerbating an existing disease. It is also understood that an unhealthy body can lead to mental problems. Often, fixing a problem in one area can help a problem in another.

After all, the brain is just another organ in the body and, while its location isolates it from the other organs, it operates on the same biochemical principals as every other part of the body. Furthermore on a cellular level, our feelings are experienced as a complex interaction of electrical signals and bio-chemical responses governed by the brain. An imbalance in mind-body interaction often results in depression. In a case of clinical depression, an imbalance of electrical signals and bio-chemical responses will make other serious diseases dramatically worse in a very insidious way. For example, it has been shown that a patient with heart disease is four to six times more likely to die of cardio-vascular abnormalities if depression is a factor.

At a 2003 national conference in Washington, DC the Depression and Bipolar Support Alliance (DBSA) revealed that scientists have made great strides in understanding the underlying causes of depression and are attributing them to a defect in a combination of key genes and triggers within the patient's living environment. This is why depression often runs in families. Also, women are twice as likely to become depressed than men, although men are less likely than women to admit their depression.

There are roughly 60 electrical bio-chemicals circulating in the brain known as neurotransmitters that transfer messages between cells. Studies have shown that serotonin is one of these essential neurotransmitters that circulates everywhere throughout the body, not just in the brain. It is believed that many of the neurotransmitters involved in the physiology of clinical depression can have negative effects throughout the body when they become imbalanced, disrupted, or diminished.

According to the Institute of Natural Resources, there are three primary neurotransmitters believed to be involved in depression: norepinephrine, dopamine, and serotonin. Studies show people with depression have diminished levels of these neurotransmitters.

Purposed Associated Disorders of Three Common Neurotransmitters

Norepinephrine (noradrenaline) is associated with motivation, energy, socialization, appetite, arousal, alertness, and basal metabolic rate. An imbalance of norepinephrine is also associated with diseases such as various forms of depression disorders and autonomic nervous system disorders.

Dopamine is associated with concentration, socialization, hunger, sexual desire, motor control, pleasure, and reward. An imbalance in dopamine is associated with depression, schizophrenia, Parkinson's disease, and ADHD.

Serotonin is associated with mood, emotions, appetite, food intake regulation, limbic system functions, pain, and sleep. An imbalance of serotonin is associated with depression, anxiety, appetite disorders, and migraine headaches.

The Monoamine Hypothesis

Norepinephrine, dopamine, and serotonin are the three neurotransmitters known as the "neuroamine triad," which forms the basis for the "monoamine hypothesis." The monoamine hypothesis proposes that depression results from the under-activity of the neuroamine triad within the central nervous system.

The limbic system and the hypothalamus are two parts of the brain that are extremely sensitive to changes in the balance of neurotransmitters. The limbic system is responsible for controlling moods, behaviors, and emotions; the hypothalamus is responsible for elevated levels of cortisol, controlling the pituitary gland's production and release of hormones, and regulating thirst, hunger, and temperature. Neurological disorders such as Parkinson's, epilepsy, Alzheimer's, and stroke involve physical alterations in the brain, including the death of cells responsible for producing dopamine, which is crucial to movement control and mood. When clinical depression accompanies these disorders, drugs that work on improving serotonin chemistry do not always help in relieving the patient's depression because these drugs do not help with the production of dopamine. In Parkinson's disease, the physical alteration of the brain organ itself not only affects its ability to produce dopamine, it also affects its ability to produce other neurotransmitters, such as serotonin, norepinephrine, and glutamic acid, all of which are involved in different forms of depression.

Three Classes of Drug Therapy For Depression

1) Selective Serotonin Reuptake Inhibitors (SSRIs): Repairing the bio-electrochemical imbalance occurring in depression is the aim of all treatments for depression. The first class of drugs aimed at treating depression is called selective serotonin reuptake inhibitors (SSRIs), such as Prozac, Zoloft, Luvox, Paxil, and Lexipro. SSRIs are single reuptake inhibitors, working solely on keeping an even serotonin level in the bloodstream. They do this by impeding the quick reuptake (slowing absorption) of the monoamine enzyme serotonin into nerve cells, so serotonin levels remain balanced in the synaptic cleft (the area between two nerve cells where a club shaped nerve fiber almost touches another nerve cell in order to transmit a signal) after serotonin is secreted from the presynaptic cells.

2) Tricyclics: A second class of drugs aimed at restoring neurotransmitterbalance is tricyclics, such as Elavil, Amitril, Tofranil, and Cymbalta.

Tricyclics are dual reuptake inhibitors that impede the reuptake process of the monoamine enzymes serotonin and norephinephrine so these monoamines at the synaptic cleft remain active for longer periods of time. When an SSRI does not seem to work, a tricyclic may.

3) Monoamine Oxidase Inhibitors: A third class of drugs aimed at treating depression is monoamine oxidase inhibitors (MAOIs), such as Marplan, Nardil, and Parnate. MAOIs are triple reuptake inhibitors that are used for only a small number of people. MAOIs inhibit the activity of the enzyme monoamine oxidase, particularly subtypes A and B, which play a role in metabolizing serotonin, norepinephrine, and dopamine by preventing all three of these neurotransmitters from breaking down.

With any of these drugs, side affects such as intense sleepiness, dizziness, and blurred vision can occur. When these drugs do not help depression, electroconvulsive therapy (ECT), also known as low voltage shock treatment, can reset the electrochemical state of a depressed brain. This therapy has been very successful in patients whose depression was not being helped by drugs.

The brain chemistry of a patient can also be very effectively adjusted with talk-therapy, especially when it is used in conjunction with medication and other therapies. Talk therapy includes cognitive therapy, where the patient learns to recognize destructive patterns in their lives and develops practical ways to break bad mental habits. Also, the use of biofeedback can relieve stress and lower cortisol levels in the body. By learning to control the way you think and respond you can actually change your own biochemistry.

Researchers have only just begun unraveling the exact interplay between depression and disease, although there is already strong statistical evidence linking depression to many diseases such as Epilepsy, Alzheimer's, Parkinson's disease, fibromyalgia and stroke. It has also been scientifically proven that rebalancing the biochemistry of depression may reduce the deadly impact of severe disease. Since the average doctor visit is ten to fifteen minutes long, the subject of depression is not always explored.

A patient should always go into the doctor's office with a list of issues they wish to address, including how they are feeling psychologically, even though they may be seeing a specialist in another field. It is also wise to keep in mind that tweaking the biochemical levels of the brain through the use of SSRIs, tricyclics or MAOIs, can produce dangerous side effects. When dealing specifically with the relationship between depression and fibromyalgia, you have to consider the relationship between depression and pain. In 2003, Dr. Schatzberg, MD led a study at

Stanford University that revealed a strong link between depression and chronic pain. Dr. Schatzberg stated, "People who have major depression are more than twice as likely to have chronic pain when compared to people who have no symptoms of depression."

Schatzberg's Observations Linking Depression and Chronic Pain

- All kinds of pain (mild, moderate, or severe) co-exist with depression.
- Depression is a strong and independent predictor for debilitating neck and low back pain.
- Depressed patients with back pain use twice the sick days and have higher health care costs than patients who only have either pain or depression, but not both.
- Depression complicates treatments for back, neck, and chronic pain.
- Persistent pain is commonly associated with post-traumatic stress disorder (PTSD) symptoms among patients with chronic headaches.
- 43% of patients with depression have chronic pain.
- 20% of chronic back pain patients have unipolar major depression (UMD).
- For patients experiencing both depression and pain, medications aimed at reducing both depression and pain symptoms are the most effective.

To further understand the relationship between depression and chronic pain, it is also important to look at the role serotonin plays. A 2004 study by Doctors Crowell, Jones, and Harris suggests that serotonin plays a major role in depression, chronic pain, and in visceral pain syndromes that occur with the stretching and contracting of gastrointestinal organs (irritable bowel syndrome). Antidepressants, such as SSRIs and tricyclics, work with the neurotransmitter serotonin because serotonin is important in both the central and enteric (intestinal) nervous systems.

Low serotonin levels in the synaptic cleft contribute to a biochemical imbalance in the brain. Because such an imbalance causes depression, and depression causes pain, decreased levels of serotonin lead to depression and pain. Antidepressants that balance serotonin levels can effectively treat pain and depression by preventing the quick re-uptake of serotonin in the brain and prolonging the time serotonin is present in the synaptic cleft.

Depression Does Not Account for All FMS Symptoms

The pain syndromes that are caused by depression have all been documented in scientific studies. Even so, the fact remains that these clinical depression related syndromes do not completely account for the long list of symptoms that fall under the umbrella of chronic fibromyalgia syndrome.

Because of this fact, I do not believe that depression alone can be considered a cause of chronic FMS. Treating depression with an antidepressant is likely to relieve the depression that subsequently occurs with FMS; however, FMS cannot be reversed by treated depression alone. FMS patients must realize the importance of treated depression, and what role their depression plays in their illness, but must also realize that antidepressants alone are not going to cure them.

Furthermore, the depression from FMS naturally creates anxiety that can become chronic. Chronic anxiety creates the high cortisol and adrenalin levels of the fight or flight response. Chronic anxiety also creates the bio-chemical imbalances that cause depression to become chronic, and chronic depression creates more pain. It is a never-ending vicious cycle. But hang in there with me. There are plenty of ways to improve your condition while you are curing it, and I will outline them all in the following chapter.

Phoenix Rising

Out of the pyre of life's injustices, from events unearned and unforeseen,
Emerges a caged and broken spirit, now injected with the power of
immortal love
It ascends like a shining phoenix out of its rival darkness
With a blast of comet-like force and so furious a will that drives its
blazing wings
As streaks of light glow wide beneath
The phoenix rises and breaks free, illuminating all that has gone before
In a single flash of comprehension, never to sink or descend again
The ignited intention from its recovered power surges within the heart of
Its reclaimed spirit, coursing through miles of electric veins
As the magnificent phoenix rises again as once before
When as its truest, most incandescent self was unfettered by event
or time
Brilliant with love and consciousness
On fire with its natural blinding luminosity
You, the phoenix, return.

Valerie Lumley

Phoenix: An ancient mythological bird resembling an eagle that lived for
500 years, and then burned itself to death on a pyre from whose ashes
another phoenix arose.

Chapter Six
Theories of Physical Causes

When considering the origins of disease, it is always profitable to reflect on past theories that have lasted throughout the ages and stood the test of time. The famous 16th Century physician and alchemist Paracelsus, also known as "the pathfinder" and "father of modern medicine," made numerous references to spiritual causes of disease in his Volumen Paramirum. He said, "The human body has been constructed from out the wisdom of the entire cosmos: The salt, sulfur and mercury composing the body cannot cause disease, this is solely due to the influences brought to bear on it by the human soul, as bearer of the Ego."

Paracelsus goes on to say about all who are the alchemists of their own lives, "Should the alchemist not be capable of separating (at the right time) that which is healthy from that which is poisonous, then do good and bad remain together, and the process of putrefaction runs its course. And what is more, this process goes forward at the expense of the entire organism, for a parasitical life comes into being and all material life, escaping the energies of the alchemist, becomes parasitical life within the human body – it creates disturbances and the result is illness."

Paracelsus seems to be addressing the position of today's scientific community, which says the majority of the body's cells are bacterial. This profound imbalance between bacterial cells and the body's own cells impacts the human body and its overall health. Furthermore, when he refers to separating, at the right time, that which is healthy from that which is not, I believe he is including physical injuries to the body that also affect the soul in "poisonous" ways. Physical injuries, if not properly handled, can cause chronic illness.

Injuries to the body that are substantial enough to result in chronic illness can be as minute as an invasive organism or as major as a serious accident or assault. When a physical injury occurs, the damage it may do to the soul can be just as profound; both spiritual and physical injuries can negatively impact one's body and one's wellbeing. Because of this, both the mental and the physical wellbeing of a patient must be addressed in treatment.

Paracelsus also asserted that "The causes of disturbances to the organism have their origin in disturbances affecting the soul's life, and that sicknesses are the materialized results of injuries done to the soul. Thus, passing on from incarnation to incarnation do the soul's faults of today crystallize into the bodily ailments of tomorrow – into the next life's tendencies to this or that disease. Now, as ever, is the spirit the builder and the architect of the body. Reason can make it an object of study and experiment, and may, as the direct results of such study and research, propound that system of hypothesis, known as the Science of Medicine. Yet, as to the secret of that balance so imperative between the soul of today and the body of today – these are matters whereof modern medical science knows nothing."

Within these lines Paracelsus seems to allude to what science now calls inherited personality and disease tendencies in the DNA, which can be passed to new generations from previous ones. He refers to the origins of these disease tendencies as "injuries to the soul" that have been brought forward from a previous life through the phenomenon of reincarnation. According to this belief system, experiences brought forward from a previous life would fall into the category of "karma" which, among other things, deals with what may be called "unfinished business." Paracelsus also refers to general injuries to the soul that eventually materialize or manifest as disease.

This assertion is aligned with the fundamental Christian Science belief that thought materializes itself. Again, the injuries to the soul and the thought patterns that surround them do not address physical injuries to the body, which cause subsequent injuries to the soul, a detail which seems to be missing from current medical practice.

Currently, chronic FMS is thought to be caused by the aforementioned injuries to the soul and resulting psychological disorders and pathologies. One of my doctors attended a seminar in southern California in 2004 which asserted the theory that, "A great many patients with chronic FMS suffer from Borderline Personality Disorder."

In his "Volumen Paramirum," Paracelsus talks about the sages and the "divine knowledge" they possessed regarding the secret of balance between body and soul, "A balance which, be it observed, differs according to the people and the tribe." Certain habits and customs still drifted on beyond the middle ages, but in time those ties were severed. The loss of this connection to ancient habits and customs led us to find our own. Whereas people used to eat and drink to survive, today we eat and drink what we choose. The value of sustenance as a sustainer of life and an energy source has been overshadowed by the value of the pleasure derived from food that tastes good. This has resulted in weak bodies and subsequent disease. What a difference between the self-will of today and the forceful "thou shalt" or "thou shalt not" of the Mosaic Law.

As Paracelsus asserted, how we live our lives and what we put into our bodies certainly has a direct effect on our health, and I think we all know this. We have so many choices concerning our health that taking responsibility for it can be very difficult. A patient with chronic FMS can no more ignore what they put into their body than someone who wants to float on a barge in piranha infested waters can ignore the fact that it is being held together with twine. Your liveliness is literally at stake and you have to pay very close attention to what you choose to consume.

General Theories of Physical Causes

1) The Four Pillars of Reversing Chronic Fibromyalgia

The Transfer Factor, Volume I — Infectious Diseases, follows a case of chronic FMS. The publication refers to a theory called "The 4 pillars (or foundations) in reversing fibromyalgia." These "pillars" are: nutrition, exercise, stress management, and supplements. Transfer Factor, a manufacturer of supplements, sells an entire line of nutritional supplements formulated specifically for people suffering from FMS.

Therapeutic nutrition is an extremely important aspect in treating FMS, as is stress management and gentle exercise. I would say that these "four pillars" are essential factors in reversing or healing chronic FMS, but I do not believe they alone represent the full means to a cure, or that a lack of proper nutrition is a cause of FMS. Adding a nutritional protocol to your treatment combination will help you feel stronger and will give you more energy; however, supplementing your diet with the proper vitamins will not cure the condition.

2) The Three-Factor Theory

Another theory about the cause of chronic FMS is the "three factor theory." According to this theory, FMS is caused by a combination of three factors, which are stress, chemical and toxic elements of our environment, and trauma.

Toxins are a concern to everyone, especially someone who is very ill, but not everyone who has stress and who is exposed to toxins has chronic FMS. Therefore, the third factor of this theory seems to be of utmost importance for this theory to work. Studies have shown that a trauma often triggers the onset of chronic FMS. Usually, the trauma is minor and compounds earlier injuries. According to the "three factor theory," the trauma can be physical, psychological, or emotional.

Specific Theories of Physical Causes

1) Omega-6 Aracidonic Cascade Into PGE2

This theory involves post-traumatic chronic pain after an injury. The "Omega-6 Arachidonic Cascade Into PGE2" involves the acceleration of the catabolism (conversion) of omega-6 trans fatty acid (TFA) arachidonic acid into pro-inflammatory prostaglandin E2 (PGE2), resulting from tissue inflammation. This inflammation produces a variety of local biochemical events causing hyperexcitability of the CNS, synaptogenesis/ neuroplacsticity of the spinal cord (neuropathic pain with profound plasticity changes), and receptor field enlargement (body-wide pain).

It begins with a trauma that releases the inflammatory mediator "tumor necrosis factor alpha" (TNF-alpha), which activates the enzyme phospholipase A2, which liberates arachidonic acid from the cell membranes. This increases the production of pro-inflammatory mediators PGE2, leukotrienes (LTB4), and nitric oxide (NO). Inflammatory mediators TNF-alpha, PGE2, and NO all add to adjacent nerve fiber injury, causing neurological dysfunction, excessive muscle tension, spasms, and pain.

Pro-infammatory PGE2 also increases the firing of the sympathetic nervous system (SNS), causing vasoconstriction and immuno-supression. This immuno-supression causes the destruction of T-cells resulting in many systemic health issues, particularly cancer. Studies have shown that people who suffer from chronic pain have up to a 200% increased risk of dying from cancer. Although the only cervical spine trauma referred to as a basis for this theory is whiplash, I believe any trauma or series of compounding injuries to the cervical spine, and other cervical maladies, can result in various forms of cervical myopathy (chronic muscle spasms and/or pain in the cervical spine) and have a potential for causing chronic body-wide pain.

The process resulting in the phenomenon of chronic-pain called the omega-6 arachidonic cascade into PGE2 occurs subsequently to cervical spine trauma as follows: a) Trauma to the cervical spine causes tissue damage, which is not recognizable through available diagnostic methods; b) The absence of evidence does not mean that there is no tissue damage; c) Tissue damage produces inflammation that is primarily caused by the Arachidonic Cascade.

An article in the Division of Inflammatation and Pain Research, Los Angeles Pain Clinic 2007, vol. 69, pp. 1169-1178, Medical Hypothesis of Inflammatory Pain, describes inflammatory pain transmitted through the nociceptive afferent system. There are two afferent systems that mediate external and internal pain and sensation to the central nervous system and brain, called the nociceptive and the non-nociceptive afferent systems. The nociceptive afferent system transmits pain, while the non-nociceptive afferent system transmits non-pain sensations.

According to this article, nociceptive pain is caused by the peripheral tissue release of inflammatory mediators prostaglandins PGE-2, leukotrienes (LTB4), and nitric oxide (NO), and is characterized by somatic and visceral nociceptive pain. Somatic pain tends to be localized, constant pain that is sharp, aching, throbbing, or gnawing. Visceral pain tends to be vague in its distribution, spasmodic, and described as deep, aching, squeezing, and colicky in nature.

Four Effects of The Arachidonic Cascade

- It alters the thresholds of the nociceptive afferent system (the nerves that carry pain impulses from the outer body to the brain and/or spinal cord) and may also activate normally inactive nociceptors, increasing pain.
- It causes a specific gene expression in the dorsal root ganglion (a structure containing a dense cluster of nerve cells at the bottom of the brain), which results in an increased peripheral receptor field, or "receptor field enlargement" (meaning the pain experienced at the site of the trauma is widened to include a larger area in the body and can even spread to body-wide pain).
- It accelerates the conversion of omega-6 TFA into PGE2 by increasing the production of cyclo-oxygenase-2 (COX-2) in the spinal cord (an enzyme that converts the omega-6 TFA into PGE2). This results in increased production of PGE2, which results in neuronal hyper-excitability and more pain.
- The increase in production of COX-2 expressed in the spinal cord and supraspinal centers alters the experience of pain sensitivity in the entire body, causing hypersensitivity to spread to non-injured areas.

All of the above biochemical responses induce profound changes in spinal cord plasticity (ability to bend or mold). This is called adverse, maladaptive central nociceptive synaptogenesis/neuroplasticity (neuropathic pain syndrome with profound spinal plasticity changes or "stiff spine"). These biochemical responses to cervical spine trauma cause injury to the spinal disc and facet joints, which are the most probable sources for the initiation of the perception of chronic pain.

Injury to disc and facet joints causes nearby spinal segments to involuntarily contract, resulting in a decrease in the range of motion. This reduction in movement opens the pain gates and accelerates disc and facet joint degeneration (early degenerative disc disease). All of these changes result in increased pain that can persist after all potential tissue healing has occurred. In a reported 10% of cases, these changes can be irreversible, causing a chronic pain syndrome.

The conversion of omega-6 trans fatty acid into PGE2 causes many problems, including: inflammation; stiff and dysfunctional cell membranes; and the alteration of protein receptor shapes, which alters the way in which your body reacts to neurotransmitters, hormones, polypeptides, and amino acids. The result is the physiological alteration of the cell membrane and the expression of cellular DNA. Unfortunately, omega-6 fatty acids are present in many sources of food. American culture is full of foods that contain the fatty acid; trying to maintain a diet low in omega -6 fatty acid is crucial.

In addition, a stiff and dysfunctional cell membrane alters the ability of ions to cross over the membrane, causing arrhythmias (irregularity in normal rhythm of ionic activity). Unfortunately, pharmacotherapy aimed at inhibiting the Omega-6 Arachidonic Cascade into PGE2 has been related to fatal GI bleeding, liver damage, kidney damage, and rebound alterations of receptor sensitivity, such as severe headaches. Furthermore, the Arachidonic Cascade is accelerated by the use of antibiotics and refined carbohydrates, which trigger the production and release of insulin.

Happily, the generous ingestion of omega-3 essential fatty acid (EFA) inhibits the process of the Omega-6 Arachidonic Cascade into PGE2, but should not be taken unless you also take double bond antioxidant factors. In 2002, 2003, and 2004 research has provided objective proof that patients with chronic pain have reduction of movement and plasticity changes in the spinal cord, hypersensitivity of the spinal cord neurons, increased risk of dying from cancer, and lasting chronic pain beyond all possible tissue healing that has occurred.

2) Activity Dependent Neuroplasticity

An article from *Biomedical Science*, issued by the University of California at Riverside, discusses evidence supporting trauma to the neck as a cause for chronic central nervous system sensitization and chronic pain in motor vehicle collision victims and patients with fibromyalgia. In this article, "activity dependent neuroplasticity" is described in both acute and chronic pain hyperalgesia (excessive sensitivity to pain) as pain due to a continuous generation of nerve pain mediators (nociceptors) caused by damaged tissue. Activity dependent neuroplasticity also causes profound plasticity changes and stiffness of the spine causing hypersensitivity of the CNS.

Although several studies indicate that this small persistent input of nociceptors can lead to pain continuing after damaged tissue has healed is caused by neuroplasticity; studies also indicate that minor peripheral nerve injuries are an underestimated source of the persistent hypersensitive state of chronic pain. These injuries can include whiplash, a bump on the head, a lifting and twisting accident, compounding minor injuries, or any type of minor spinal trauma. Studies show that in trauma or inflammatory injury serotonin is released, sensitizing muscle nociceptors to the chemical and mechanical stimuli that cause muscle hyperalgesia.

Criteria for peripheral mechanisms of muscle tenderness and hyperalgesia

- There is no biochemical test that can show a measurable biochemical cause for chronic pain.
- Chronic pain is not being caused by external sensory input through the nociceptive afferent system, but is coming from neurogenic type pain cause by CNS hypersensitivity.
- Chronic muscle pain both originates in the central nervous system and is maintained by it.
- This central nervous system mechanism may explain fibromyalgia and myofascial pain syndromes.
- The weight of evidence suggests that fibromyalgia is a chronic pain syndrome that has a central rather than a peripheral or muscular basis.

Further studies as recent as 2004 and 2005 support the theory of "activity dependent neuroplasicity" in fibromyalgia after a whiplash injury from a motor vehicle collision, and site a wide variety of evidence and implication. Whiplash associated disorders carry a thirteen-fold risk for developing chronic fibromyalgia. The onset of fibromyalgia syndrome is significantly associated with trauma in the preceding six months. The evidence that the trauma of motor vehicle collision may trigger fibromyalgia meets established criteria for determining its cause.

The Canadian Clinical Working Case Definition, Diagnosis, and Treatment Protocols from 2003 states, "There is strong consistency in documentation that physical trauma such as a fall or motor vehicle accident, particularly a whiplash or spinal injury, can trigger fibromyalgia in some patients." These studies, in addition to all the presentations of plausible etiological mechanisms (causal mechanisms) make a compelling argument that trauma to the neck or spine does in fact play an etiological role in the development of chronic FMS in some, but not all, patients.

A review of whiplash type injuries to the neck and spine indicates that most minor injuries will heal in two to three months and that 25% will become chronic. This study also states that injuries involving the discs, the zygapophysial joints, or the alar-ligaments will not resolve spontaneously and usually become chronic. These patients are likely to improve for up to two years and not beyond two years; however, I would like to point out the latter conclusion was made by a researcher who viewed this study through the lens of his own scope of knowledge and, like all specialists, this view can be biased and should not necessarily be taken as fact. The body is designed to heal itself and, if given the right help and support, this healing mechanism should continue to function for the duration of the life of the body, not for a maximum of two years.

All of these studies and treatment protocols discuss the phenomenon of a long-term increase in the exitability of neurons in the spinal cord, and generalized central hypersensitivity, suggesting changes in central pain processing mechanisms. These factors can cause exaggerated pain following low intensity nociceptive peripheral stimulation in whiplash victims and patients with fibromyalgia where pain is absent of detectable tissue damage. While blocking pain pathways in sufferers of acute pain may work, because of the nature of chronic pain this line of treatment is not effective.

If you have read this far, by now your brain may feel tired and your eyes may feel crossed. Even if all you have done is skim through this data, you have most likely acquired a clear understanding that dozens and dozens of articles and studies over more than a decade so far have all alluded to the same thing: a trauma to the neck and spine, even some kinds of minor compounding traumas, can trigger the chronic pain of fibromyalgia and all its ill effects.

A Comprehensive Overview of Chronic Pain Phenomena

Before leaving the discussion about the biochemistry of chronic pain, I think it would be beneficial to review some of the important points. An article from a seminar in southern California in 2002 regarding chronic neuromuscular pain states the term "neuromuscular pain" has become widely used in the process of diagnosing chronic fibromyalgia.

This general category has been defined to include all non-articular pain disorders that exist, despite treatment, for longer than six months and display regional and palliative factors consistent with abnormalities arising in myofascial tissue, such as in myofascial pain syndrome. This category also considers the relationship between the sympathetic nervous system and chronic pain originating in or near muscular connective tissues having the characteristics of sympathetically mediated or neuropathic pain.

This article addressed the pathophysiologic mechanisms underlying chronic neuromuscular pain and describes several syndromes that can be categorized under this general term.

Pathophysiology of Chronic Neuromuscular Pain

- Disturbances in the transmission of pain signals from the body's periphery (through the nociceptive and non-nociceptive afferent systems) to the central nervous system that lead to central sensitization, the phenomena of "wind-up" and "centralized pain."
- Neuroendocrine abnormalities.
- Abnormalities of regional cerebral blood flow to the thalamus of the brain.

Nociception

Beginning with changes or disturbances in the nociceptive afferent system, nociception is a neurochemical process by which a pain signal is transmitted from the periphery of the outer-body to the central nervous system of the inner body and mediated by A-delta and C-nerve fibers located in skin, bone, connective tissue, muscle, and viscera. Pain signals travel from the periphery along primary afferent neurons, which synapse in the dorsal horn of the spinal cord and continue on into the thalamus (a pair of egg-shaped masses of gray matter lying beneath each cerebral hemisphere of the brain).

From the thalamus these signals travel to the cerebral cortex (the wrinkled outer layer of the frontal parts of the brain responsible for sensation perceptions), resulting in the perception of pain. The nociceptive process begins with a noxious stimulus, such as a trauma or injury, that distorts or damages tissue. Such trauma then leads to the arachidonic cascade.

Other chemical byproducts produced by tissue damage and inflammation include prostanoids and serotonin. These chemicals activate neurons in the dorsal horn of the spinal cord, which leads to the release of elevated levels of excitatory amino acids that stimulate the nociceptive neurons and cause an on-going sensation of pain.

Pain is modulated in two systems: the ascending pain modulation system and the descending pain inhibitory system. Serotonin and norepinephrine are two of the predominant neurotransmitters in the systems.

The ascending pain modulation system originates in the midbrain and projects to the thalamus beneath each cerebral hemisphere through serotonergic fibers.

The descending pain inhibitory system has several fibers that modulate the transmission of nociceptive signals through spinal neurons to supra-spinal structures from endogenous (originating within a tissue) antinociceptive systems. When stimulated, these systems work together to modify pain sensation and inhibit behavioral reactions provoked by injury or trauma. The spinal mediators involved in descending pain inhibitors are the neurotransmitters serotonin, norepinephrine, and acetylcholine.

Central Sensitization/Hyperexcitability of the CSN

When central sensitization, or CSN hyperexcitability, of the nervous system occurs, it is a result of an injury or trauma that stimulates muscle afferent-C fibers. This causes excitatory amino acids and peptide neurotransmitters to be released in greater amounts and for an extended period of time.

If the afferent-C fibers are stimulated for too long, normally silent interspinal synapses may be activated, leading to the sensitization of second-order spinal neurons. Prolonged stimulation can also result in the activation of neurons that are located some distance away from the initial trauma, causing pain to become widespread.

Receptor Field Enlargement

Receptor field enlargement widens and prolongs the perception of pain and causes it to be more intense. After second-order spinal neurons have become chronically sensitized, the result is body-wide allodynia and hyperalgesia, when all sensations are experienced as pain. What was formerly a non-painful sensation becomes a painful one, and what was formerly a painful sensation becomes even more painful.

Central Pain

The phenomenon of central pain occurs when non-nociceptive afferent neurons act on a sensitized CNS. Central pain has been defined as, "the experience of pain produced by the excitation of non-nociceptive neurons or the excitation of nerve fibers that normally relay non-painful sensations to the spinal cord."

Four mechanisms in the pathophysiology of central pain

- Central sensitization induced by past or on-going nociception.
- Convergence of both nociceptive and non-nociceptive afferent neurons onto the same secondary neurons in the area of spinal cord called the dorsal horn.
- The experience of pain from a low level of neuron stimulation.
- An exaggerated pain response extending beyond the initial area of injury.

Four defining characteristics in Non-nociceptive (or neuropathic) Pain

- The description of pain seems inappropriate when compared to the degree of tissue pathology.
- Trauma results in hyperalgesia, or a pain experience that is more severe than would normally be expected.
- Normally non-noxious stimuli, such as a light touch, result in pain.
- The pain extends beyond the location of the trauma.

Wind-up

Wind-up occurs when repetitive stimulation activates unmyelated C fibers, which leads to a cumulative increase in discharge of second-order neurons in the spinal cord. This increase in second-order activity leads to the progressive build-up in magnitude of electrical responses recorded in the dorsal horn of the spinal cord.

The wind-up phenomenon explains how the persistent stimulation of a peripheral nerve can lead to the hyperexcitability of the CNS, causing hyperalgesia, allodynia, persistent pain, and receptor field enlargement. In fibromyalgia, this is experienced as chronic pain.

Sympathetically Mediated Pain

Sympathetically mediated pain is described as severe pain, usually of a burning quality, associated with minor soft-tissue or peripheral nerve trauma followed by changes in the autonomic nervous system. The autonomic nervous system controls our involuntary functions, such as heartbeat and glandular secretions. Autonomic changes can involve symptoms such as abnormal sweating or vasomotor instability (instability in the diameter of blood vessels). When this kind of pain follows a nonspecific local injury to bone or soft tissue it is called complex regional pain syndrome Type 1.

In this syndrome, initial nociceptive impulses are transmitted through nerve fibers to the dorsal horn, where they stimulate neurons that become sensitized and more responsive to all subsequent afferent system stimuli. This causes hypersensitivity which, along with associated changes in the sympathetic nervous system, is dependent on levels of norepinephrine, one of the neurotransmitter associated with pain perception. The other is serotonin. Sympathetically mediated pain is also associated with other chronic pain syndromes, such as myofascial pain syndrome (MPS), chronic fibromyalgia syndrome (CFS), and chronic tension-type headaches (TTH). Because of this, and the association of pain with the central nervous system, an effective treatment would have to maintain a healthy balance in nervous system activity, rather than just mask the symptom of pain.

An example of such a medication is a dual reuptake inhibitor, such as Cymbalta, a relatively new drug that balances levels of norepinephrine and serotonin. Triple reuptake inhibitors, or MAOIs, are available but are not generally recommended, as they can be dangerous. Triple reuptake inhibitors control levels of norepinephrine, serotonin, and acetylcholine.

3) Kidney Malfunction

The theory of a genetic kidney malfunction as being the cause of fibromyalgia has become well known, thanks to R. Paul St. Amand, MD's 1999 publication, *What Your Doctor May Not Tell You About Fibromyalgia*. His book is well written, his theory is very well thought out and I believe there is truth in his observations that a certain aspect of kidney malfunction manifests its effects in the body in a way that coincides with various FMS symptoms; however, I do not believe that kidney malfunction is the cause of FMS. I believe it is only one of the symptoms of FMS.

Dr. St. Amamd's book talks about a genetic malfunction in the kidneys which causes them to re-circulate an excess level of metabolized calcium phosphates back into the bloodstream. The kidneys are supposed to re-circulate some calcium phosphates, but an excess of them will accumulate in the soft tissues, theoretically causing muscle spasms and pain. A build up of calcium phosphates then prevents the cell matrixes from producing normal levels of energy (ATP), resulting in chronic fatigue and causing the cascade of other chronic FMS symptoms.

Dr. St. Amand's recommended treatment uses a form of generic guaifenesin found in Musinex, an over-the-counter allergy medicine intended to liquefy mucous, which also removes excess calcium phosphates from the body. I felt this treatment protocol had some merit so I tried it for two years. The treatment made me feel instantly worse, but over time I do believe that I felt better; however, the benefits of the treatment fell short of providing a cure.

Kidney malfunction may be one of the many symptoms of FMS, but not its cause. Although Dr. Amand's intentions are good, his observations are made through the lens of his specialty, and as such may fail to see the bigger picture. Mistaking a symptom as a cause is not unusual in the medical world.

This is missing the medical boat and, unless all doctors become familiarized with the overall nature of chronic FMS, its diagnostic criteria, and its overall symptomatology, this mishap will continue to occur. It is also likely that focusing on treating the most predominant symptom, usually with suppressive drugs, will cause the fibromyalgic to get worse overall. This happens because the body is struggling to maintain a sense of balance and the delicate tight-rope the body is walking can be easily disrupted by outside interference of any kind, including medical treatment. In fact, almost any type of symptom management treatment given to a fibromyalgic often makes their pain worse for a time, and rarely helps overall.

As with other helpful protocols, such as nutrition, stress reduction, and gentle exercise, it is typical among fibromyalgics to see some improvement, but then level off short of being 100% cured. I do recommend his book for reference and educational purposes, and I do acknowledge the testimonials he relays about patients who have experienced profound improvements with his protocol. However, my personal experience has shown me that this protocol is not the last word in completely abolishing chronic FMS.

4) Hippocampus Malfunction

A September 4, 2008 article published online at PubMed from the Department of Family-Medicine, LSU Health Sciences Center, Shreveport, Louisiana asserts the theory that metabolite abnormalities in the hippocampus of the brain may be responsible for symptoms in chronic FMS. The article states, "A growing body of evidence suggests involvement of the central nervous system in the poorly understood pathology of chronic FMS." I cannot help but think of the sarcasm "No shit, Sherlock!" However, I promise to refrain from making such comments as we move forward (bad writer!).

After all, the scientific community is required to measure and prove everything in a tangible way before making any statements that might be subjected to scrutiny. This is good to bear in mind when you come across articles or studies about breaking news in the area of FMS science.

What the scientific world must prove through tests and experiments I know through first hand experience. I love Dr. Albert Einstein for saying, "True knowledge only comes through experience." Believing in what you know through experience is something we as patients have the right, the responsibility, and the luxury to do.

The hippocampus, like the hypothalamus, is the part of the brain associated with the storage of our memories and is very sensitive to stress. The adverse affects of stress on the hippocampus can be seen in patients who suffer from Alzheimer's disease. When under severe or chronic stress, the condition of these patients worsens. A sudden shock can cause them to dramatically advance in the degeneration process of their memory centers. The aforementioned article asserts that the hippocampus is adversely affected in a variety of disorders, including chronic FMS, whose onset is associated with a trauma, which is a stressful experience.

The article talks about a case-control study using a small control group of premenopausal female FMS patients who met the American College of Rheumatology criteria for FMS classification, an age-matched group of healthy females, and a single-vowel proton magnetic resonance spectroscopy (PMRS), which measures hippocampus metabolites. A single vowel (a three-dimensional unit of video screen imaging) was placed over the right hippocampus area of the brain.

The tests demonstrated a significant reduction in the hippocampal metabolites ratio of N-acetylaspartate to creatine (NAA/Cr ratio) in the right temporal lobe of the brain in patients with FMS. In addition, there was a significant negative correlation made between FMS patient scores on the Fibromyalgia Impact Questionnaire (FIQ) showing aspects of cognition, depression, sleep symptoms, and the low metabolite ratios shown on the PMRS test results. These combined results indicate that brain metabolite abnormalities are associated with FMS.

The report states, "We have demonstrated an abnormality in hippocampal brain metabolites in premenopausal female fibromyalgia patients with **no** psychiatric comorbidity (appearance of multiple pathologies). A significant negative correlation between patient subjective experience of symptoms and a reduced NAA/Cr ratio suggests a role for hippocampal pathology in fibromyalgia."

This conclusion makes it clear that a trauma can cause a malfunction in the hippocampus and that this does not indicate the existence of a psychological illness. In fact, this conclusion indicates psychological trauma that is not a result of a psychological illness is sufficient to cause a malfunction in the production of hippocampal metabolites.

However, this does not rule out the possibility that psychological illness can exist prior to the onset of FMS. This means that, although a psychological illness may not be sufficient stress to cause FMS, the stress of such an illness will certainly contribute to the severity of chronic FMS symptoms. Furthermore, when there is an emotional and/or physical injury to the central nervous system that affects the brain, this can involve the following three inter-related systems.

Three inter-related systems of the brain involved in CNS trauma

- The limbic system – the primitive part of the brain where suffering and stress is experienced.
- The hippocampus – the part of brain where memories are stored.
- The hypothalamus – the part of the brain that regulates all autonomic functions of the body, including arousal, blood flow, body temperature, hormonal balance, and also stores memories.

The hippocampus secretes a pain messenger called substance P, the secretion of which can become accelerated under stress. Also secreted under stressful conditions are adrenaline and cortisol, both of which are released by the HPA Axis, which is a system made up of the hypothalamus, the pituitary gland, and the adrenal glands. In FMS patients, the brain, especially the hippocampus, becomes very delicate and vulnerable to the affects of stress, even to the point of atrophy. Traumatic emotional and/or physical injuries involving the CNS have been proven to adversely affect all of the above and add to the severity of FMS symptoms.

Another study in 2008 involving hippocampal metabolites done by the Department of Rheumatology and Rehabilitation of Cairo University in Cairo, Egypt used the same criterion for control groups to observe the correlation between FMS patients and hippocampal metabolite ratios (NAA, chorine, and creatine) in both the left and right hippocampi. Like the aforementioned study they used a single-voxel proton magnetic resonance spectroscopy (PMRS). FMS patients and healthy controls underwent psychological testing to assess cognitive function, depression, and sleep.

The study also included a Fibromyalgia Impact Questionnaire (FIQ), a test for the number of tender points and a visual analog scale (VAS) for pain. Their published conclusion with regard to theory of cause for FMS states, "NAA levels of right and left hippocampi differed significantly between patients and controls. The hippocampus was dysfunctional in patients with FMS as shown by lower NAA (N-acetylaspartate) levels compared to controls, representing neuronal or axonal metabolic dysfunction. As the hippocampus plays a crucial role in maintenance of cognitive functions, sleep regulation and pain perception, we suggest that metabolic dysfunction of the hippocampus may be implicated in the appearance of these symptoms associated with this puzzling syndrome."

Both studies conclude hippocampal dysfunction may explain a few symptoms in fibromyalgia syndrome based on results using single-voxel PMRS. Although the first study hypothesizes a trauma of some kind might be responsible for its dysfunction, both studies fall short of proving a cause for FMS because hippocampal dysfunction accounts for only a few of its symptoms. Once again it seems a symptom of chronic FMS (the dysfunction of the hippocampus) is being singled out as a possible cause.

While stress worsens all FMS symptoms and very likely plays a significant role in the malfunction of the hippocampus, there are still a wide variety of malfunctions throughout the body's physiology that are not explained by the hippocampal metabolite abnormalities found in these studies. Therefore, a hippocampal dysfunction is clearly more likely to be a symptom of FMS and not the cause.

5) Hypothalamus Malfunction

In 2006 a Glasgow author by the name of Dr. David Mickel wrote a book called *Chronic Fatigue Syndrome* and went on to develop what he calls the "Mickel Therapy" for treating fibromyalgia. His theory of cause is FMS patients have unacknowledged or unresolved messages and emotions between the body and brain, causing a "split" between what the body knows and what the brain is saying.

Dr. Mickel says, "There is an emotional reality that is at odds with what your head is thinking and this causes a build up of activity in the mid-brain. Because these emotions go unresolved over a long time, the hypothalamus goes into overdrive and gets stuck. In CFS and FMS the "switch-off" mechanism stops, and it keeps going." He goes on to say since the hypothalamus is responsible for regulating every physiological part of the body, a chronic state of hypothalamic overdrive would cause the entire body to overwork in every way on a 24/7 basis. In his theory, this explains a majority of FMS symptoms.

Dr. Mickel has coined the phrase "body intelligence," which refers to what are commonly called "gut instincts." Body intelligence can create emotions just as thought can, and trumps the brain's intelligence in terms of importance. I like this idea, as it aligns with my previous thoughts about the importance of maintaining an internal alignment between your gut instincts and your thoughts.

I support the importance of this idea because I fully understand through experience how energetically draining it is for your body and your mind to be at odds. Your body/mind intelligence simply must be aligned for your life-force energy to resonate fully throughout your body.

Mickel Therapy is simple; Dr. Mickel teaches FMS patients to listen to their bodies and learn to understand, acknowledge, and honor the messages the body is sending to the brain. He explains that the body does not respond to positive affirmations the way the brain does, and that the body creates its own emotions and sends them to the brain in the form of symptoms when its messages are not being acknowledged.

Dr. Mickel uses a three step technique to teach patients to decipher, "If the body could speak, instead of sending symptoms, what would it being saying, what was the body unhappy about at that time?" The result of his remarkable therapy is that 92% of his patients got better. As the unacknowledged emotions and messages from the body were brought into the foreground and dealt with properly, the hypothalamus regained normal function and overall symptoms improved.

Dr. Mickel's remarkable "Three Keys To Health"

- Define yourself energetically, meaning when the body feels unfairly treated, you just won't take anymore.
- Develop how you are able to express the feelings that are being created in that moment as a "facilitator."
- Bear in mind the "key to self." When the body knows that the self is a priority, it will send less emotional energy to the brain.

I love this method of helping people recondition themselves by having them put their own wellbeing before that of others. Even in an airplane you are asked to put your oxygen mask on before helping others. Part of the importance of putting yourself first is that you will be able to help those around you when they need it.

I applaud Dr. Mickel for his success in helping FMS patients get better and teaching them how to live in a healthier way. This is wonderful. If you would like to learn more about his work, go to www.mickeltherapy.com, where you will find written and video records to peruse and enjoy. He is a delightful man and a wonderful asset to alternative health methods. Although Dr. Mickel's approach has not yet been studied, I feel it has great merit toward overall improvement. I also believe hypothalamus malfunctions would certainly be aggravated by an internal incongruence between body and mind intelligence and the stress this causes. However, I do not believe it is enough to cause chronic FMS.

Not everyone who is misaligned between their body and the mind intelligence has FMS and I see this theory as another case where a symptom of FMS has been misidentified as a cause. All of these theories are like spokes on a giant wheel branching out from the same center, separate from one another but connected. The outside band of the wheel is the manifestation of chronic full-blown FMS and the center is what is called the Atlas subluxation.

6) Spinal Stenosis/Atlas Subluxation/Cervical Myopathy

Spinal stenosis occurs when a person is born with an abnormally small opening in the foramen magnum (the opening at the base of the skull through which the spinal cord passes from the medulla oblongata of the brain into the vertebrae of the spine), or develops a narrowing of this opening throughout his or her life. Spinal stenosis can eventually cause chronic FMS on its own or it can contribute to suddenly triggering the onset of chronic FMS with the help of a major or minor compounding neck injury.

Theoretically, spinal stenosis surgery is said to alleviate chronic FMS symptoms by surgically making the opening larger and relieving the pressure that is put on the spinal cord, but the results of this surgery are not guaranteed. I personally know a man with chronic FMS who, after being bedridden for ten years, opted to undergo this procedure. He was diagnosed with spinal stenosis and told he would be "a new man" in two to three months after the operation.

His chronic FMS was triggered by a minor neck injury while golfing, however the misalignment of his Atlas cervical vertebra (C-1) was never detected by the chiropractor. Sadly, the predicted outcome of the surgery was not realized. Immediately after the surgery he experienced a worsening of his condition for a period of several months and again became bedridden. It took roughly one and a half years before he began to experience a marginal benefit from the surgery, and years later he is still struggling with disabling FMS symptoms. Eventually, with my recommendation, he got his Atlas checked and a two to three millimeter misalignment of his Atlas vertebra was detected.

One of my former doctors told me about another woman who had chronic FMS who also had this surgery in hopes of reversing her condition. After her surgery she, too, experienced a profound increase in the severity of her symptoms, became bedridden from increased pain, and was unable to move her body or turn her head without experiencing extreme dizziness and nausea. I was also told she did not improve for a very long time and had sued her surgeon. In spite of my former doctor's warning, she was desperate enough to go ahead with the surgery.

I do not know what the statistics are of reversing chronic FMS with this particular surgery; however, if you are born with a small opening of the foramen magnum there is absolutely no room for even a one or two millimeter misalignment of the Atlas (C-1) vertebra without experiencing the onset of FMS symptoms. I would suggest you get your Atlas vertebra checked by an upper cervical spine Chiropractor before you consider an invasive procedure and that you only consider surgery as a last resort.

7) Brain Stem Injuries

Brain stem injuries can occur from a wide variety of traumas, most commonly whiplash from an automobile accident, and become chronic over time. The brain stem is made up of three parts: a lower part, a middle part, and an upper part.

- The lower part called the Myelencephalon (medulla oblongata) balances and calms the nervous system and brain activity to allow sleep.
- The middle part called the Metenchelphalon (pons) is the fibrous tissue connecting the lower and upper parts of the brain stem.
- The upper part called the Mesoencephalon (mid-brain) stimulates brain activity, the firing of the autonomic and sympathetic nervous systems, the hypothalamus, and the production of hormones in the pituitary and adrenal glands.

The brain stem enters the spinal chord at the base of the skull in the back of the head through the "Foramen Magnum" (Greek for large hole). It travels from the center of the brain through the Atlas (C-1) vertebra and becomes the spinal cord (cervical, thoracic, lumbar and sacral spine). An Atlas subluxation pinches the brain stem where it becomes the spinal cord and causes a brain-stem injury that becomes chronic over time if the misaligned Atlas is not adjusted back into 100% alignment.

A brain stem injury causes the over-firing of the upper brain stem, which hyper-activates the central nervous system (CNS) and above related parts of the brain, resulting in the hyper-sensitization of the entire CNS. The lower part of the brain stem becomes inhibited and unable to adequately balance and calm the over-firing upper part, and the result is an imbalance of hormone production and the inability to sleep. When ongoing cortisol (the stress hormone) is produced by over-stimulated adrenals, the "fight or flight" syndrome becomes chronic which causes the degeneration of brain cells (gray matter). The result is the toxic, body-wide bio-chemical environment responsible for the brain-fog and body-wide symptoms of chronic fibromyalgia syndrome.

Thirty-five years ago I was involved in a serious automobile accident on a rainy night in Los Angeles, California on my way to Mexico. I was riding in a Volkswagen bus in the passenger seat, asleep with my head resting on a pillow, and I was wearing my seat belt. All of a sudden a semi-truck pulling two open trailers of sand came barreling down an on-ramp onto the freeway in a hurry to get ahead of the pack of traffic about 100 yards behind us. He was not looking at what was on the road in front of him, did not see our bus, and plowed straight into the side of the front part of the sliding door behind my head. My seat belt caught me as the blow sent me flying to the left toward the dashboard and windshield.

The truck driver struggled to free his front bumper, which had become wedged behind my head between the back of the passenger seat and the sliding door. Finally, the front bumper broke off his truck as he jack-knifed to the right, causing his two trailers to overturn. As he tried to slow his rig down we gently pulled to the left and managed not to turn over. I could see out my passenger window his two trailers on their sides spilling sand on the freeway as the sides of the metal containers were dragged along the road throwing six-foot sparks in every direction. At this point in the accident I was in and out on consciousness and bleeding profusely from the back of my head.

The pack of traffic behind us saw the sparks and slammed on their breaks in an attempt to avoid the sand and two overturned containers. As we pulled over to the inside left shoulder I could see the cars on the wet slippery freeway as they were crashing into each other and piling up to the right. It was horrific. I lost consciousness until one of six ambulances arrived. An ambulance technician opened my door and carried me into his nearby vehicle. The right side of the back of my head had been split open about two inches and had bled out onto my sweater and pillow. I was still bleeding in the ambulance while the paramedics attended my head wound.

I remember saying to him, "You have a hard job. I guess you're pretty used to this kind of thing by now." He looked at me with such compassion and love in his eyes and said, "Little lady, the day I get used to this is the day I quit." I will never forget him. I arrived at the emergency ward of a nearby hospital and was helped into an exam area by the paramedic. I was briefly examined, stitched up by an uninterested nurse who was gossiping with the other nurse across the ward, and released without any further tests. There was nowhere to go to recover and rest so my friend and I ended up continuing our journey to Mexico, where my friend took out my stitches on a beach two weeks later.

I have told this story to every doctor I have seen since the onset of my FMS in 1993. All of this was repeatedly dismissed with relatively no interest and was never given the attention it was due. I felt this accident had a significant, if not crucial bearing on why a subsequent compounding and relatively minor injury had triggered my full-blown condition 22 years after it had occurred.

Just prior to the onset of my chronic FMS I had sustained a compounding neck injury doing crunches at home on the floor. I was crunching to the left and reaching my right elbow toward my left knee when I felt a small pop at the top of my neck and a pain shoot down the right side of my back. My back became increasingly tight and, in two week's time, I was unable to move.

From that day on I experienced a steady increase in symptoms rendered me completely bed-ridden in three short years. It took ten more years and over a dozen doctors before I received an accurate FMS diagnosis.

I finally found my way to a local Osteopath who was the first to palpate the top of my neck and verify that I had a notably severe misalignment of the Atlas vertebra, so I asked him for a referral to a local chiropractor that could do the adjustment.

Now that I was in the care of two doctors who were willing to pay attention to my theory and work with me, I felt I could really begin to make some headway in healing this illness. The chiropractor I began seeing was wonderful; he listened carefully to my story, palpated my neck, confirmed significant misalignment, rotation, and tilt of the Atlas vertebra, and adjusted it, along with the compensating cervical vertebra misalignments, on the first visit. He stated in fifteen years he had never seen an Atlas/C-1 vertebra that was as far out of alignment, "shifted a half a thumb to the left, with rotation and tilt." He began a conservative alignment protocol to correct the misalignments in my Atlas, my neck, and my upper back, which had been strained and misaligned due to compensation stress from the Atlas misalignment.

There are numerous ways the Atlas can be misaligned, such as a left or right shift, a left or right rotation, a left or right tilt, or a forward or back shift. The forward shift is the misalignment that can become locked into place and requires a special kind of adjustment. When symptoms persist after adjusting the other misalignments, it usually means that there is a forward shift that has become locked in place and is the final adjustment that needs to be made. This can be detected through a simple x-ray down the throat.

When I saw my first x-rays they confirmed that the left lateral Atlas shift, the right Atlas rotation, and the right head tilt were results of both of my injuries. I realized this fit perfectly with my own theory and was indeed the underlying occult cause of my condition. Most importantly, I learned to trust my gut instincts; I was not a crazy psychotic, a hysterical hypochondriac, or a malingering histrionic, and FMS was not depression with somatazation.

The auto accident 22 years prior to the onset of the FMS had offset my Atlas to the left, but not enough to trigger the onset of full-blown chronic FMS. My strong body, youthful vitality, innate strength, and determination were able to compensate for the effects of the initial misalignment. However, the minor compounding neck injury while exercising at home 22 years later was the straw that broke the camel's back. This injury had further popped the Atlas out in the same direction and triggered the onset of chronic, full-blown FMS. The C-1 subluxation had created an on-going brainstem injury.

As I entered into my new chiropractor's conservative treatment plan, he was very hesitant to adjust my neck too often in fear of making my delicate condition worse. Even though I began to improve immediately, my Atlas kept shifting laterally to the left between adjustments, but not as far. This caused my symptoms to ebb and flow. I was improving overall, but because the muscles and tendons holding the Atlas in place have memory and had become stretched out for so long, they wanted to go back into the old position and were not strong enough to hold the new one.

Consequently, the Atlas would continue to slip between each adjustment, resulting in my being unable to completely heal. I went on this way for a couple of years, grateful for the increase in my activities of daily living (ADLs) but still very limited in what I could do.

Shortly after I began my treatment a friend told me she knew an RN who worked at Seattle Grace Hospital in Seattle, Washington. The RN had told her the doctors at the hospital were all saying that the cause for chronic FMS was cervical myopathy, which is a general term referring to muscle pain in the cervical spine area of the neck caused by various maladies such as: subluxations in the vertebrae; arthritis; disc problems; bone spurs, spinal stenosis, and so on. This was another sign of encouragement that I was on the right track; however, the generality of this term left many details unknown.

One day another friend from South Lake Tahoe, CA came to visit me and brought me an article from a local newspaper about a chiropractor who had opened a fibromyalgia relief clinic. The article said, "Chiropractor reports recovery rate of 95 percent for fibromyalgia patients." With great interest I read the article and low and behold his success was based on his Atlas alignment treatment protocol. He had found that all of his FMS patients had a severely displaced Atlas, caused by various types of trauma to the neck, such as whiplash, a blow to the head, a lifting accident, or general anesthesia causing the unsupported Atlas to slip out during surgery, and many other ways.

I was amazed to find how aggressive his treatment protocol was since my doctor had been so careful not to be too aggressive in fear of making me worse. I then decided to step up my treatment protocol with my chiropractor to one adjustment per day until my Atlas began holding at 100%, then decreasing the frequency of my visits according to how well my Atlas would hold. He was game to try it so we went for it. The South Lake Tahoe doctor's more aggressive approach gave me the confidence to become more aggressive in mine and his reported success further confirmed my belief all along that the misalignment of my Atlas had been the cause of my condition. I knew aligning the Atlas was the key to healing this disease and this would be the beginning of my complete recovery that would allow the subsequent brainstem injury to heal.

According to the South Lake Tahoe doctor, when the Atlas vertebra is not 100% in alignment, it puts pressure on the spinal cord at the top of the neck where it meets the brain stem at an opening at the base of the skull, called the foramen magnum. It also puts torque on the membrane that surrounds and protects the brain and spinal cord that contains the cerebral-spinal fluid, called the meninges. The spine serves as Grand Central Station for the central nervous system and all the grand nerve trunks of the body enter into the spine between the vertebrae from outside the spinal cord though attachments along the meninges.

Because the tissue of the meninges is fibrous and inflexible, when pressure from a misaligned Atlas is inflicted on it at the base of the skull, it tugs on all of the nerve trunks up and down the entire spinal column. This causes the nerves to fire at an abnormally high frequency, resulting in impulses to and from the brain to become distorted. The brain receives and interprets these distorted impulses as an abnormal or unexplained pain, burning, itching, numbness, tingling, pricking sensations on the skin, and much more.

This soon causes acute aggravation, hyperaction and sensitization of the entire central nervous system. Both the sympathetic and autonomic nervous system pathways become overwhelmed, resulting in chronic, severe body-wide dysfunction and pain.

It seems the cure for chronic FMS can be as simple as aligning the Atlas vertebra 100% and the subsequent compensative subluxations, strengthening the stretched out connective tissues that hold the Atlas in place and rehabilitating the body. In my case, I discovered this kind of

100% alignment was not resulting from the periodical adjustments of my chronically misaligned Atlas; however, I decided not to partake in the more aggressive approach.

I believed that the doctor from South Lake Tahoe was on the right track because I had already experienced a degree of improvement from my own chiropractor's more conservative Atlas alignment protocol. After careful consideration, I felt the best course of action was to develop my own, more moderate treatment plan.

Furthermore, I knew my insurance company would consider this treatment plan experimental unless I could prove medical necessity. If I stayed with my own doctor, I could do this by contrasting previous progress with the accelerated progress of the new treatment.

Comprehensive Overview of the Atlas Subluxation

The anatomy of the Atlas (C-1 at the top of the spine) subluxation in its articulation to the Occiput (C-0 at the back of the head where the skull joins the top of the spine) and its articulation to the Axis vertebra (C-2 beneath the Atlas) is a phenomenon that has been theorized among many to account for a vast majority of human illnesses. This is because of the devastating affect this misalignment has on the brainstem, spinal cord, the central nervous system, and the musculoskeletal system. The Atlas subluxation is also known as the Grostic Kink Subluxation, which is a term that honors Dr. John F. Grostic and his 1946 publication, *The Chiropractors Field Research Manual.*

Interestingly, John Grostic was diagnosed with Hodgkin's disease in his early twenties by a doctor who gave him only two years to live. Instead of accepting this fate, Mr. Grostic decided to go to a chiropractor in the office building where he worked. He was treated and then referred to the B. J. Palmer research clinic in Davenport, Iowa, where he received upper cervical care and made a full recovery. After an accidental neck injury prompted a relapse of Hodgkin's disease, Mr. Grostic returned for another round of treatment and, again, made a full recovery.

After his recovery, young Mr. Grostic decided to enroll at Palmer College of Chiropractic and graduated in 1933. He began his intensive research into the analysis and correction of the occipito-atlanto-axial subluxation, developed the Grostic procedure, and taught from 1946 until his death in 1964. Dr. Grostic specialized what he called Chiropractic Orthospinology (Greek words *orthos* [straight] + *spino* [spinal column] + ology [science or branch of study]). After many years of research, Dr. Grostic concluded that "the only true subluxation—vertebral misalignment with nerve interference—occurred in the upper cervical spine" and the only adjustment given at his famous clinic was in the occipito-atlanto-axial area.

To quote a 2006 article from the *Academy of National Upper Cervical Chiropractic Association (NUCCA)* regarding the effects of the Atlas subluxation, "The nerve insult mechanism is hypothesized as traction on the central nervous system via the supporting system of ligaments, specially the first denticulate projection at the foramen magnum, when the occipito-atlanto-axial segments are out of alignment." This traction (or torque) on the spine, brainstem and affecting the central nervous system comes from the kink in the spinal cord at the top of the neck, which is caused by Atlas subluxation.

The brain stem and spinal cord exit the brain through the foramen magnum, which is a hole at the base of the skull. The spinal cord then travels through the opening of the Atlas vertebra and down into and through to the tip of the spinal column, which is made up of twenty-four cervical, thoracic, and lumbar vertebrae. Between the vertebrae are twenty-three discs that serve as shock absorbers for the spine (there is no disc between the Occiput and the Atlas it sits on).

The spinal cord sends signals from the brainstem through the body via the central nervous system meant to regulate all biological systems, movement, sensations, and healing. From the central nervous system (CNS), these messages travel through the great nerve trunks, which exit the vertebrae along the meninges.

These great nerve trunks divide into a smaller and smaller network of nerves that fan out and permeate the entire body, much like veins and arteries divide into smaller and smaller blood vessels and capillaries. The body's network of nerves makes up the central nervous system just as the body's network of blood vessels makes up the circulatory system.

These are very delicate and complex systems and the body cannot be healthy without both of them functioning properly. For the CNS to function properly, the Occiput must be perfectly aligned with the Atlas vertebra to avoid any torque on the meninges or compression or kinking of the spinal cord, cervical nerves, and blood vessels that wind their way through the neck. Any torque on or compression of these structures would interfere with the brain's signals to and from the body and the circulation of oxygenated blood to the brain.

The Neck is a Busy Place

To understand the phenomena of the Atlas subluxation it is important to understand all that is going on in the neck itself, with regard to biological systems. The neck houses just about everything but the kitchen sink. Most importantly, it includes the part of the central nervous system where the brainstem joins the spinal cord at the top of the neck and the cervical nerves that join the central nervous system network. It also houses the circulatory system, including the carotid arteries and the jugular veins, the musculoskeletal system, including the cervical vertebrae and all the muscles and ligaments surrounding and supporting them, the respiratory system, including the larynx and main bronchial tube between the nose and mouth and the lungs, and, finally, the digestive system, including the tongue and the esophagus between the mouth and the stomach.

Aside from these obvious aspects of the neck there is also the human skull, which weighs as much as a bowling ball. If the center of gravity of the bowling ball is shifted even slightly, the ramifications to the entire body can be devastating. Imagine holding up a bowling ball at the top of your wrist when it is balanced and when it is not. When it is not, holding it for long it will cause pain and strain to your fingers, wrist, elbow, arm muscles, shoulder, and eventually your neck, back, and the rest of your body.

To understand the full effects of an Atlas subluxation it is essential to understand the anatomy of the C-1 vertebra itself and its relationship to surrounding structures. To begin with, the C-0 (occiput) occipital condyles (the two rounded ends of the base of the back of the skull) sit on top of the superior articular condylar surface of the C-1 (Atlas) vertebra below it. The Atlas sits on top of the C-2 (Axis) vertebra below it. The Atlas is what is called a double condyloid joint, meaning that at each outer side of the vertebra are rounded edges protruding left and right from its center where the C-O condyles sit.

In the 1977 publication of Gray's Anatomy, by Henry Gray, details about the Atlas are found on pages 229-331: "This articulation is a double condyloid joint. Its ligaments are the Anterior Occipito-Atlantal, the Posterior Occipito-Atlantal, two Lateral Occipito-Atlantal, and two Capsular-Atlantal ligaments." The spinal cord and spinal nerves can be seen in cadavers as being tethered by these tiny ligaments to the inner margins of the vertebral foramen (the holes of the vertebrae through which the spinal cord travels). On each side of the Posterior Occipito-Atlantal ligament there is a passage to allow the penetration of the first cervical nerve and the vertebral arteries.

The route of these vertebral arteries exits through the foramen in the transverse processes of the Atlas and penetrates the Posterior Occipito-Atlantal ligament before it loops up into the brain. There are many other ligaments and muscles supporting the heavy skull and brain, attaching it to the cervical spine that enables movement such as twisting, bending, and rotating. These are tiny ligaments representing key structures of the musculoskeletal system existing in and around the Atlas vertebra and cervical spine.

Other key structures in and around the connective tissues of the Atlas are four pairs of major cranial nerves. These nerves are called the Vegus, the Spinal Accessory, the Glossopharyngeal, and the Hypoglossal nerves. Underlying the Sternocleidomastoid muscles are the well-known Carotid arteries and the Jugular veins. There are also large, deep muscles at the base of the neck and at the junction of the shoulders called the Scalene muscles. These muscles are divided into three groups called the Posterior, the Medial, and the Anterior Scalene muscles. It is important to note the origin of the vertebral arteries where they divide from the subclavian arteries (underneath the collarbone) and the brachial plexus of nerves are in very close proximity to the Anterior Scalene muscle.

When there is a subluxation of the Atlas at the top of the neck both the vertebral arteries and the brachial plexus of nerves can become seriously compressed by the muscles of the head and neck as they strain to maintain the upright position of the skull on top of the cervical spine. This compression (or traction) can also adversely affect the Phrenic nerve that runs between the Anterior and Middle Scalene muscles on its way to the diaphragm.

When the Atlas is properly aligned, the normal anatomy is for the occipital condyles of the skull to sit perfectly on top of the condylar surfaces of the Atlas, and for the lateral masses of the Atlas to sit on top of the facet joints of the Axis vertebra below it. The posterior Odontoid Dens that upwardly protrudes from the middle of the Axis vertebra is seated centrally inside the Atlas, toward the foramen magnum. When a traumatic force is delivered with enough force to the left side of the skull, for example, the skull is pushed sideways and the Odontoid Dens slides along the condylar surface of the Atlas to the left.

The occipital condyles of the skull can slide off center relative to the Atlas condylar surface, resulting in a left head tilt with the Atlas positioned high or elevated on the right, and the Axis Dens no longer positioned centrally to the foramen magnum. It is important to note that the ligaments of the neck limit this over and/or under lapping. Furthermore, the anatomy of the Atlas with regard to the slope of its condyles will determine if the Atlas will rotate in its relationship to the occiput above. If the slope of the Atlas condyles is steep, it will reduce a great deal of potential rotation; whereas if the surface of the condyles is flat, rotation can be present in a subluxation as well as a lateral shift.

Tension in the muscles and ligaments of the neck caused by the Atlas subluxation in their effort to hold the head upright can have drastic effects on the spinal cord. This subluxation can also have drastic effects on the vertebral arteries traveling through the cervical spine from C-6 and up to the Atlas, on the Carotid arteries, which travel underneath the Sternocleidomastoid muscles and up through the foramen magnum into the brain, and on the cranial nerves that leave the foramen magnum at the base of the skull and wind down through the neck.

All of these structures can be kinked, pinched, stretched, trapped, tugged on, and otherwise compressed by the resultant narrowing of the opening between the foramen magnum in its articulation to the displaced Atlas, and the Atlas foramen in its articulation to the Axis, and by the chronic tension of the muscles and ligaments of the neck as they struggle to hold the head upright. The result of the effects of this strain is a reduction in blood flow and the weakening and distortion of cranial nerve signals to and from the brain involving the Vagus nerve, the Spinal Accessory, the Hypoglossal and the Glosopharygeal nerves of the cervical spine.

The health and function of the body relies upon the nerves of the central nervous system and the arteries of the circulatory system to be in optimum working order; when they are not the entire body suffers. In fact, with an Atlas subluxation, the many muscles and tiny ligaments in the sub-occipital region of the cervical spine and the larger muscles and ligaments of the neck become so severely stressed that they spasm, resulting in a kinked spinal cord at the craniocervical junction.

This causes stress and irritation of the neurological and vascular structures at this junction and throughout the cervical spine. The structures in close proximity to the muscles and ligaments being stressed, such as the vertebral arteries and the cranial nerves that exit the Posterior Occipito-atlantal ligament, are especially vulnerable to these effects.

For instance, as the Greater Occipital Nerve (GON) exits the spine at the C-2 it travels along a tortuous course through a number of cervical muscles on its way up the cervical spine to the Occiput, and is particularly vulnerable to compression from the spasms of the cervical tissues. The GON wraps around the Obliquus Capitus Inferior muscle, travels toward the skull, pierces the Semispinalis muscle, and then pierces the Trapezius muscle at the Occiput. Along this course this nerve can become impinged and/or entrapped at one or all of these locations, creating pain and headache symptoms that increase in severity and frequency with ongoing occipital nerve irritation. This results in the migraines frequently experienced with this subluxation.

The muscles and ligaments affected the most by an Atlas subluxation are the Rectus Capitus Posterior Minor and Major, the Obliquus Capitis Superior and Inferior, the Sternocleidomastoid, the Leveator Scapula, the Trapezius, and the Anterior and Posterior Scalene muscles. When these tissues become painful, the act of simply holding up your head seems impossible. These tissues, especially the Trapezius muscles, can become so painful, the only relief found comes in laying the head down in a prone position and taking all of the weight off the top of the neck.

This is why people with a serious Atlas subluxation end up spending so much of their time in bed. Over time, the muscles and ligaments of the neck and shoulders begin to atrophy, causing more pain and disability. In addition to realigning the Atlas, the muscles and ligaments of the neck and shoulders will require rehabilitation, as they will need to build back their strength.

In addition to headaches, neck and shoulder pain, and the atrophy of neck and shoulder muscles and ligaments, there are further adverse effects of the Atlas subluxation that must be fully understood. Severe Atlas subluxation can cause unbearable pain that starts in the head, neck, and shoulders and radiates throughout the body. An Atlas subluxation that is minor may only result in periodic headaches, low back pain and other minor biological disturbances.

The Myodural Bridge

In a 1995 issue of *Spine Magazine*, Dr. Gary D. Hack, D.D.S. wrote an article about a major breakthrough in the anatomy of the cervical spine called, "Anatomic relationship between the Rectus Capitus Posterior Minor muscle (RCPMI) and the Dura Matter." The article discusses a study that discovered a previously unknown ligament that directly attaches the posterior arch of the Atlas vertebra to the pain-sensitive Dura Matter of the brainstem and cerebellum. The attachment of the RCPMI to the Dura Matter at the base of the skull has since then become known as the Myodural Bridge. This article proves a direct connection between this ligament and the central nervous system.

In all eleven cadavers examined in this study, this tiny structure of dense connective tissue was discovered to connect the RCPMI muscle to the Posterior Atlanto-Occipital membrane, "that was fused to the Spinal Dura by numerous fine connective tissue elements." Since the joints of the upper cervical spine are rich in proprioceptors that provide positive feedback to the brain, it is a fact that any subluxation of the Atlas vertebra will result in traction of the Dura Matter of the central system.

Studies have shown this traction causes the distortion of feedback to the brain, along with chronic headaches, migraines, dizziness, and balance disorders, such as Menier's disease, especially since this misalignment goes hand in hand with the atrophy of the sub-occipital cervical muscles. Studies have also shown that a correction in the Atlas alignment by an upper cervical spine chiropractor has reversed the symptoms of Menier's disease.

The Dura Matter (Latin for "tough mother") is the outermost, toughest, and most fibrous membrane of the brain and spinal cord, and is like a thin layer of strong cellophane. This layer is bathed in spinal fluid that is held in by the meninges. It continues down through the base of the skull into the spine, connecting the vertebrae, discs, and muscles surrounding the spinal cord, and enclosing the cerebrospinal fluid around the brain and spine. It also wraps around and protects the great nerve trunks that exit the spine.

The Dura Matter's sheath is composed of two partially fused layers and an outer layer, called the periosteum. Located between these layers are the sinus veins and the trigeminal ganglion, which connect to the fifth cranial nerve (nervus trigeminus). The layer of Dura Matter connected to the spinal cord is called the spinalis and is separated from the periosteum by a space containing blood vessels and fibrous and areolar tissues.

Researchers at the Michigan State University College of Osteopathic Medicine suggest, "The function of the Rectus Capitus Posterior Minor (RCPMI) muscle is to provide static and dynamic proprioceptive feedback to the CNS, monitoring movement of the head, and influencing movement of the surrounding musculature." The RCPMI muscle is now considered to be more of a "sensory organ" than a muscle which arises by a narrow pointed tendon from a tubercle on the posterior arch of the Atlas, winds up in ascension and inserts itself into the medial part of the Inferior Nuchal Line at the back of the occipital bone, into the surfaces of the occiput and the foramen magnum, attaching to the spinal Dura (CNS).

In November of 2008, a newsletter published in "Chiropractic Health & Wellness" by Warren Hammer, CD, MS of Norwalk, Connecticut describes what he called The Dural Connection. The article states, "The Dura Matter connects the occiput to the sacrococcygeal complex and has firm osseous (bony) attachments at the entire circumference of the foramen magnum to the posterior bodies of the second and third cervical vertebrae, and within the sacral canal at the level of the second sacral segment at its anterior portion where the subdural space ends."

Hammer goes on to say, "The Dura Matter also has connections to the Posterior Longitudinal ligament. The Dura encloses the cerebrospinal fluid. The spinal nerves as they exit the vertebral foramen are covered by prolongations of the Dural sheath which blend into the paravertebral fascia." He further states that "Restrictions of motion at the occiput, sacrococcygeal complex, or at the posterior bodies of the second or third cervical vertebrae explain a significant clinical relationship between upper cervical, head and lower back pain."

This newly discovered direct connection between occipital muscles (RCPMI) and the dorsal spinal Dura has significantly broadened our understanding of the affects of the Atlas subluxation on the body. It is now a known fact that both the Rectus Capitis Posterior Minor muscle and the

Posterior Atlanto-Occipital membranes attach to the occipital bone from the posterior arch of the Atlas vertebra.

Tension of the RCPMI muscles causes a dual restriction of the pain sensitive Dura. It also causes cervical headaches and CNS our entire body by adversely influencing the flow of the cerebrospinal fluid. This has been shown in tests conducted by Dr.'s Vincent and Carmel Esposito, who worked with Dr. DaMadeian, inventor of the MRI, on the effects of spinal adjustments on cerebrospinal fluid. Together they showed a stasis of cerebrospinal fluid after a lateral subluxation of the Atlas vertebra and, in only one minute after the Atlas was adjusted and realigned, there was a significant increase in flow.

The Rectus Capitus Posterior Muscle and the Obliquus Capitis muscles are key to keeping everything in line. These "connective tissue bridges" have been proven to exist between the Atlanto-occipital junction to the RCPMI muscle and the Dorsal Spinal Dura. Furthermore, the anatomical structures innervated by the cervical nerves in C-1 through C-3 include the joint complexes of the upper three segments of the cervical spine, the dura matter, and the spinal cord. The dura-muscular/dura-ligamentous connection in the upper cervical spine and occipital area is now referred to as the Myodural Connection and involves a branch of the dorsal primary division of the suboccipital nerve.

Further effects of the Atlas subluxation are: tilting of the head; tightening of muscles along the affected side of the body; and the subsequent upward shift in the pelvis, creating what is called a "functional short leg" (as opposed to an anatomical short leg). For example, if the Atlas is shifted to the left, the head will be tilted to the right and the subsequent symptoms will be predominately on the right side of the body.

The affected side of the body will experience chronic spasms and tightening of muscles from the top of the neck, down the back and leg. In an effort to align the pelvis, the brain will initiate pelvic lift on one side of the body, causing the spinal column to twist into scoliosis and chronic contractions in the back, and creates trigger points at the bends.

This creates trigger points throughout the body. There are documented cases where the adjustment and realignment of the Atlas subluxation in patients with scoliosis has reversed their symptoms. The result of these one-sided symptoms will soon lead to problems with degenerative hip and knee, ankle, groin, and calf problems. The chronic flexion of one side of the body also creates compensative problems on the other side of the body. The compression of key cervical nerves manifests in every kind of pain and dysfunction imaginable throughout the body, including restless leg syndrome.

The Atlas Subluxation Accounts For the Unique Symptoms of FMS

All of the symptoms developed and uniquely presented by each FMS patient are accounted for in the effects of the Atlas subluxation. Because of the weight of the skull and the elasticity of its ligaments, a traumatic blow to the head may drive and jam the Atlas in one direction or another. The combination of symptoms that each patient develops depends on the individual's anatomy and the direction and amplitude of the force of the trauma received.

Daniel O. Clark, D.C. illustrates the effects of the Atlas subluxation on his website at www.uppercervicalillustrations.com. His illustrations clearly show how this injury causes severe imbalance throughout the body. Based upon my personal experience, I believe the cause of chronic fibromyalgia to be head and upper cervical spine trauma resulting in the Atlas subluxation, subsequent subluxations, and body-wide pain and dysfunctions.

A skilled upper cervical spine chiropractor can align your Atlas and cervical spine and help you heal the brainstem, your neck, back, and body. Try to remember that everyone heals at his or her own rate and the right healing combination may vary from person to person; however, to cure chronic FMS, the cervical spine must be addressed first and foremost. The right combination of legitimate alternative therapies, gentle exercise, energy nutrition, and classical constitutional homeopathy will make you feel better, but they alone will not be curative.

I believe that if you are suffering from chronic FMS, the best thing you can do for yourself is seek out a reputable, licensed upper cervical chiropractor in your community that possesses experience and expertise in the treatment of the Atlas vertebra and cervical spine, has the capability to x-ray down the throat for an Atlas subluxation, and can diagnose your spine with special attention to C-1 through C-6 vertebrae. The kinds of cervical myopathy that can contribute to chronic FMS can come from a variety and/or combination of other conditions in the neck, in addition to the Atlas subluxation.

However, I feel the cause of chronic FMS is the misalignment of the Atlas (C-1) vertebra in its articulation with the Occiput (C-O) above and the Axis (C-2) below, the subsequent brainstem injury, and the compensative vertebral subluxations and spinal pathologies caused by trauma to the head and neck. FMS can be triggered by one injury or by a "last straw" minor injury in a series of compounding injuries. These can take many forms.

It has been my experience that the cure for chronic FMS is the realignment of the Atlas-Occipital subluxation and any subsequent compensative subluxations in the neck, back, and pelvis. There are other injuries that can cause the kind of chronic cervical myopathy that increases the severity of chronic FMS symptoms, such as: bulging discs; herniated discs; degenerative discs; bone spurs; osteoporosis; osteoarthritis; and spinal stenosis, and brain stem injury from whiplash.

When seeking treatment for chronic FMS, begin with a conservative approach. Because of the fragility of your body in this condition, talk with your chiropractor about a safe but effective treatment plan. Listen to your instincts, take charge of your treatment, and chart your progress. In 1912 D. D. Palmer became known as the father of chiropractic medicine. His son, Dr. B. J. Palmer, continued his father's work, "It is useless to administer a powder, potion, or pill to the stomach when the body needs an adjustment."

My Fibromyalgia Symptoms

My FMS symptoms began nearly four decades ago, soon after a serious car accident in which I sustained a blow to the right side of my skull that shifted the Atlas vertebra to the left. These symptoms showed up as: TMJ on the right side of my jaw; tennitis (ringing in the ears); excessive ear wax production in the right ear; gastro-intestinal problems; digestive problems; functional shortening of my right leg; right hip pain; left shoulder pain; and upper arm muscle "kinking" when I would raise it over my head. I would also occasionally experience spasms in the Longisimus muscles on the right side of my back if I twisted the wrong way.

These symptoms were not disabling; they were more like a manageable nuisance than tell-tale signs of a crippling disease. Stress worsened these symptoms of course, but they did not interfere with my life to any serious degree. I also had mental stresses that were caused by on-going problems in my life choices and in the relationships I was involved in. It was not until I experienced a compounding injury to my head and neck from improperly executing sit-ups at home that I popped the Atlas further to the left, triggering the onset of full-blown chronic FMS.

Once my FMS became severe, the symptoms became more pronounced. They were no longer manageable nuisances, these chronic symptoms included: excruciating headaches; severe neck pain; degenerative disc disease between C-4/5 and C-5/6; severe pain at T-1 and T-2 through which the brachial plexus of nerves exits the spine; frozen left shoulder one year; back pain on the right side; inability to turn my head to the left; right hip pain; functional shortening of right leg; peptic ulcer disease; stomach cramping; constipation; difficulty urinating; difficulty swallowing; right side TMJ pain and distress; cold feet and hands; and shooting pains throughout my body.

There were also "bee-stings" in my hands, feet, and toes; muscle cramping in my legs; buzzing in my back and legs along the nerve meridians; "electrical worms" throughout my leg muscles; a smoldering-hot spot on the outside skin of my left knee, which eventually lead to the deadening of the nerves in an area the size of a large orange; restless leg syndrome; restless body syndrome; sharp nerve pain throughout muscles (felt like ground glass between all the muscles in my body); burning muscles; muscle tremors; muscle convulsions; and chronic muscles spasm on the right side of my back, which were so severe they pulled out the ribs attached to T-3, T-5, T-6, and T-7 on a regular basis.

There was chronic, deep gnawing pain throughout the tissues of my back; burning hot skin all over my body, especially on my back; extreme dry and flaky skin; rashes and skin bumps on upper arms and the backs of upper legs; feeling of tight scalp; frequent migraine headaches; extreme fibro-fog (could hardly form sentences); gruesome nightmares; inability to get comfortable or sleep for more than one or two hours at a time; inability to walk; dizziness; nausea; inability to hold my head up for more than a few minutes at a time; and severe depression with thoughts of suicide.

Life as I had known it was over; I was completely disabled. I was in hell 24/7 and for the first ten years I was given no diagnosis and no hope. I alone had to find my way out of this deep, dark abyss. This non-waking nightmare that had become my life was unacceptable and I was going to do whatever was necessary to heal myself and take my life back. So, as sick as I was, I used the power of my will and pushed myself forward, out of the familiar realm of traditional medicine in search of the cure.

DESIDERATA

Max Ehrmann 1927

Go placidly amid the noise & haste, & remember what peace there
may be in silence. As far as possible without surrender be on good
terms with all persons. Speak your truth quietly & clearly; and
listen to others, even the dull & ignorant; they too have their story.
Avoid loud & aggressive persons, they are vexations to the spirit.
If you compare yourself with others, you may become vain & bitter;
for always there will be greater & lesser persons than yourself. Enjoy
your achievements as well as your plans.
Keep interested in your own career, however humble;
it is a real possession
in the changing fortunes of time.
Exercise caution in your business affairs;
for the world is full of trickery. But let this not blind you to what virtue
there is; many persons strive for high ideals;
and everywhere life is full of heroism.
Be yourself. Especially, do not feign affection.
Neither be cynical about love;
for in the face of all aridity & disenchantment it is perennial as the grass.
Take kindly the counsel of the years, gracefully surrendering the things
of youth. Nurture strength of spirit to shield you in sudden misfortune
but do not distress yourself with imaginings. Many fears are born of
fatigue & loneliness.
Beyond a wholesome discipline, be gentle with yourself.
You are a child of the universe, no less than the trees & the stars;
you have a right to be here. And whether or not it is clear to you, no
doubt the universe is unfolding as it should.
Therefore be a peace with God, whatever you conceive Him to be, and
whatever your labors & aspirations, in the noisy confusion of life keep
peace with your soul.
With all its sham, drudgery & broken dreams, it is still a beautiful
world. Be cheerful. Strive to be happy.

Chapter Seven
The Search for the Cure

Navigating the labyrinth of regular and alternative medicine to discover the right healing combination can be a daunting task, especially when you are as miserable as you are with fibromyalgia syndrome (FMS). This task can take a very long time if you are not strongly resolved to be self-guided by your own truth. Discovering the right healing combination involves a very important facet of the truth. The old saying, "the truth will make you free," or, in this case, "the truth will make you well," is not always clear or easy to understand because, in the world of chronic FMS, "the truth" varies from person to person. No one person with fibromyalgia experiences it exactly in the same way as another, in the severity and duration of their illness or in the manifestation, combination, or foremost presentation of their symptoms. If you have chronic FMS you must find your own truth. Then "your truth will make you free **and** make you well." It will become **the** determining factor in taking back your life.

Your truth is something you will have to search your soul for and, once you find it, you will have to fight for it and be completely honest about it, both with yourself and with your care providers. "That's my story and I'm stickin' to it!" You cannot deny it, fudge it, stretch it, exaggerate it, hide it, only partially acknowledge it, or manipulate the facts to match what you or others need or would like to think. You must abandon any concerns about appearances or an image of yourself that no longer exists in the present. The reality of your present condition must become your first and foremost concern. Your very life may depend on how willing you are to do just that. Have you had enough? Can you do this? Of course you can.

Discovering Your Truth

You will have to be ruthlessly honest with yourself about everything and everyone in your life, past and present, if you are to gain the skills necessary to identify, hold on to, and convey your whole truth. Then and only then will you have the strength to remain true to yourself and stand up to and reject the lies, myths, and misdirected theories about chronic FMS.

Holding your ground and maintaining your position does not entail convincing others or justifying yourself. In reality, no one can understand everything about anyone. Outside validation is unnecessary for the simple reason that adults keep their own council. While you are not required to convince others about your condition or your healing choices, it is important to have people around you who provide support. When choosing these people, consider our earlier discussion about healthy relationships and boundaries.

The root of *"evil"* as a destructive force, lies in falsehoods and untruths. The egoic self must endeavor to become a seer of the truth and join in the upward struggle, growing in a continuously upward direction. One must learn to love truth more than anything else.

To quote Paracelsus, "How many souls are there that really prefer truth, loving her a thousand times more sincerely than they do that which is sweet, consoling, and illusionary? It is easy enough to pray: 'Deliver us from evil,' but it is hard to hear: 'You yourself are this evil' and in this evil you have to endure the consequences of your own shortcomings; and from this evil none but yourself can deliver you. For the petition: 'deliver us from evil' is in truth no other than an expression of the longing of the Ego to rebuild itself—to the end that it may attain that which is the sublime, and true and the eternal within man."

Throughout his life Paracelsus dared to stare into the face of truth and was thus able to see the realities behind events. He was courageous enough to be a seer of truth and held it above all else. This is the task of every human being, to be true to themselves while observing and appreciating the order inherent in all things.

When the truth is discovered and looked squarely in the face, it usually does not appear as you may have expected, especially if you have been in the habit of avoiding it. The experience of becoming a seer of truth can be an overwhelming one. The things you discover may initially cause pain, but the experience of understanding and accepting the truth is worth the process. The pain of sadness, shock, disappointment, or even anger is a necessary part of the process of seeing, acknowledging, accepting, and embracing your truth. Do not be ashamed to cry, to experience this process in its entirety.

Paracelsus said, "Tears are a form of sulfur that resolves itself into water. This means that the life current of a person's Will, which runs its course in the process of inward combustion, here meets with an obstacle —an obstacle which the person is unable to rid himself of through thought." He goes on to explain that when a person's intellect is not able to cope with what has been presented for their cognition, their emotions heat up. In this inward process, the combustion of heat and water taking place within the body causes the substances of sulfur and mercury to "substantialize," meaning the pain is substantially relieved because it is being ejected through tears.

In the natural biochemistry of emotions, emotions are subsequent to thought. In the split second prior to a thought, a choice is made about the content and quality of that thought and a chosen meaning is assigned. The thought then creates the corresponding emotion in the body.

The body also sends emotional messages to the brain by sensing things like danger and safety, which the brain then deciphers and responds to. This extremely valuable guidance mechanism is our survival instinct at work. Some even believe that our instinct (body intelligence) is our primary intelligence and that the mind's intellect is secondary. I happen to believe they are both equally important and, when properly utilized together, it would be hard to go wrong.

In a book written by Mabel Collins called *Light On The Path,* she says, "Before the eyes can see, they must be incapable of tears." This means that the "super-sentient world," or the world of truth behind the events in life, does not reveal itself to the vision of eyes that are in the habit of weeping. In other words, to clearly be a seer of truth requires refraining from tears that cloud the vision with floods of water and demands a certain maturity, ripeness, and strength of the soul.

Things that we naturally cry about such as misfortune, disappointment, loss, wrongs or sadness, are handled more with the wisdom and grace of an adult rather than the grief of a child. To see clearly, the eyes have to be free from obscuring metaphorical tears: delusions and prejudices about certain people and things must be removed before the truth about them can be understood. Think of this like the blinders on a horse. Until the blinders are removed, the horse can only see a narrow sliver of the world. Without the blinders, and likewise, without our preconceived notions and ideas, our vision is opened up to all of the possibilities of this world, not just those that dwell within our thin sliver of reality.

When the pain of an uncontrollable emotion needs to be washed away by some release of tears, they are not of an enduring, wrenching, blinding, flooding kind, but rather like a soothing flow of water that quickly and substantially resolves the pain into accepting, incorporating a painful truth into your reality. On the other hand, the egoist with his God-denuded, inflated ego and cold self-righteous heart cannot conceive of shedding tears for any reason unless it be tears of self-pity. Neither is the egoist moved by or capable of sympathizing with anyone whose experience is foreign to his own. Do not confuse the evolved, mature soul with the un-evolved egoist. They are worlds apart in emotional maturity, consciousness, wisdom and spiritual evolution.

Paracelsus said, "Conscious man experiences the outer world: subconscious man replies to those experiences with impulses of either sympathy or antipathy (hostility), and the Ego – incarnating the experience in the form of a conception, learns how to raise itself above the same." It is in this way that the mind nourishes the soul as the Ego learns to evolve in its willing, feeling, and thinking and chooses that which is healthy over that which is not.

I have always believed that conscious and unconscious impressions of the outer world transverse each other and are registered in the Ego consciousness. In other words, although the unconscious mind delivers impulses to the conscious mind in response to an outer world stimuli, and in so doing can influence our thoughts and actions to some degree, so can the conscious mind deliver impulses (or directives) to the unconscious mind and regulate those impulses according to chosen conscious thoughts.

I believe it is a two-way street and that the unconscious mind does not have sole control over the conscious mind or our chosen behavior. I also believe that, in order for the conscious mind to follow a directive from the unconscious mind, it has to agree enough to follow through and, if the conscious mind evaluates this directive and does not agree, then the directive can be overridden.

It has been my experience that habitual unconscious responses that create unhealthy impulses in the conscious mind and body can be influenced and altered by the conscious mind of anyone who takes personal responsibility for choosing their thoughts and behavior. Grounding your thinking in your own truth and accepting it can help you do this and is a very important skill.

Like learning any new skill, all it takes is practice. When your unconscious mind wants to deliver impulses to your conscious mind that undermine the clarity of your perceptions, you can choose to disregard or dismiss them and adhere to what you have come to know as your truth. The more you dismiss outdated and destructive thought patterns, the less energy you will give them and the faster they will fade away.

Rehearsing destructive thoughts and putting them on a loop like a CNN daily news cycle will make them more deeply entrenched in your unconscious mind. Rehearse what you know is true and let it sink in deeply and eventually inappropriate thoughts will fade. This will result in an inner alignment between your conscious and your subconscious, which will resonate energetically, providing the strength you need to stand fast in your truth and heal your body.

It is from here, from this place of inner alignment, that you will become your own guide to healing yourself and reclaiming your life. Depak Chopra said, "Once you embrace uncertainty, then your intuition, your creativity, your insights and your connection to the creative powers of the universe really blossom." In other words, you may not be certain when first acknowledging and embracing your truth, but you do not need to be.

Your truth will grow, as will the feelings of freedom and peace that come from being grounded in your reality and living life true to yourself. The hope that you will eventually gain from newfound clarity, freedom, and peace will motivate you to move out of despair, passivity, and resignation. This hope will provide you with the energy you need to address all of the possible treatments for your FMS.

Bernie Siegel, MD believes there are basically three types of patients

- The actor who performs to satisfy their physicians, hoping the doctors will do all the work and the medicine won't taste too bad.
- The patient who views their illness as an escape from their problems, gives up, and consciously or unconsciously wishes to die.
- The patient who refuses to play victim, who educates himself and becomes a specialist in his own condition, wants to understand the treatment and participate in the healing process. This patient demands dignity, respect, personhood, and control no matter what the course of their disease, and grows from their experiences.

Finding your truth includes determining what kind of a patient you are. If you are reading this book you are likely someone who falls into this third category. Recognizing your patient style, aligning yourself with your own truth, surrounding yourself with supportive allies, cultivating your hope, defying stereotypes and labels, taking charge of your own health, and focusing on the good that emerges from your experiences are all necessary strategies for navigating the labyrinth of regular and alternative medicine and discovering and choosing the right healing combination for you.

Pain Management Treatments and Therapies

If you have been riding the downward spiral of an FMS chronic pain cycle into physical de-conditioning and increasing pain, weakness, and depression, you are probably ready to try one or more management options to relieve your symptoms and expedite your journey back to health. In the movie The Matrix Revolution, a character called "The Oracle" said, "We can never see past the choices we cannot understand."

In other words, to be able to see into a future that includes a vision of yourself as a healthy, happy and vital human being you must clearly understand the choices available to you. In experimenting with treatment, therapy, or protocol it is important to remember you are a one-of-a-kind being who responds to everything in your own unique way.

This means a management option that works to help one FMS patient feel better might make another feel worse and vice versa. Also, it is safe to assume that because your body is doing a high-wire balancing act with regard to maintaining life-supporting functions with a deficit in energy production and a hyper-sensitized central nervous system, any kind of treatment will be a disturbance and may affect you adversely to some degree prior to providing possible benefits.

Even a gentle, non-evasive treatment that feels good while it is being given can make you feel worse later because it has interrupted the balancing act. If you feel worse for more than a day or two, ease up on the intensity and frequency of whatever treatment you are trying and see if you are able to appreciate any benefit or gain from it on a gentler level. If not, drop it after a couple of months or so and try something else. You do not need to abuse yourself further based on the promise of possible relief from any one option.

Be gentle with yourself, use common sense, and trust your instincts. There is often a short time when you will get a little worse before you get better, but do not draw this out farther than you think is reasonable. Talk to your care provider about your condition and make sure they know just how sensitive you are and how delicate a balance your body is struggling to maintain.

When you were diagnosed with chronic FMS you were probably told it is a degenerative condition with no known cause or cure, and that prescription drug management is your only treatment option. Well, this is simply not true. However, pain management without the use of a long list of heavy prescription drugs can become one of your goals while curing this illness.

Pain management can help you feel better sooner along the path to healing completely and some of the methods you discover may become an integral part of your quest to maintain a level of optimum health. There is no reason to stop doing something that has continued benefits for enhancing your health and your quality of life, and may even lengthen it to boot. Quality of life is the final goal, anyway, and some of these options can help you maintain quality of life, boost your immune system, increase your energy, physical strength, and flexibility, and help you keep your mind sharp as a tack.

Also, there is nothing that is unnatural in this chapter except for a brief mention of one prescription drug option: a dual neurotransmitter reuptake inhibitor that balances serotonin and norepinepherine. I have found this drug can also decrease the number of extra pain receptors the brain develops to receive the bombardment of pain signals in chronic FMS. The drugs usually given in a standard pain management regime for chronic FMS are all kinds and strengths of sleeping pills, muscle relaxers, anti-inflammatory drugs, painkillers or blockers and more drugs to counteract side effects. These drugs are most likely to make you worse, cause more problems with their side effects, and hasten the downward spiral of chronic pain into disabling, physical de-conditioning and overwhelming pain, fatigue, and depression.

The best way to reverse the downward spiral of a chronic pain cycle is to break it, and there are many methods available to help you do this without having to use the above-mentioned bombardment of heavy drugs. I personally do not advocate a pain management protocol that floods your body with strong and potentially toxic chemicals.

I will offer as clear and concise a description of the available alternative pain relief and management treatments, therapies, and protocols as I can. One bit of advice: make sure the professional you consult has experience in successfully helping chronic FMS sufferers with his or her technique or method and understands the full nature of this condition.

Options for your right healing combination

1) Acupressure — The ancient Chinese art of acupressure, or "contact healing," is commonly referred to as "acupuncture without needles" and is based on the same belief system. Acupressure is the older of the two arts, and, like acupuncture, it seeks to restore a patient's health by restoring the natural flow of "chi," which is the life force energy flowing throughout the body along nerve pathways called "meridians."

Instead of using needles, acupressure uses finger and hand pressure to stimulate the release of neurotrasmitters that help to inhibit the reception and transmission of pain signals to the brain. Although acupressure can be performed simply and inexpensively by a skilled practitioner, the patient can also learn several self-administering techniques called Acu-Yoga, Do-In, and Tui Na to help control their own pain through finger pressure, massage, and body positioning.

2) Acupuncture — The 4000 year old Chinese practice of acupuncture is based on the belief that the health of the body is determined by its chi energy, the same life force flowing through the meridians of every living organism. According to this belief, a person's health depends on how strong their flow of chi is and, when their chi becomes blocked or congested, a person's health can deteriorate. Through the use of needles inserted slightly below the surface of the skin into specific points along the meridians, the chi energy is brought back into balance, blocks are opened up, and congested energy is released.

The result is relief of pain and a restoration of health. The goal is always to balance the flow of chi energy and keep it flowing strong and evenly throughout the body. Relief of pain can be experienced after only one treatment or after a series of treatments. Acupuncture is also believed to stimulate the body's production of endorphins, the body's own natural painkillers, and is completely safe with no known side effects.

3) Bio-Cranial Therapy — Bio cranial therapy is a method using gentle, minute cranial massage combined with stretching of the Dura Matter at the base of the skull. This kind of therapy is being called "higher chiropractic" in that it goes beyond adjusting the vertebral subluxations. The minute movement of the skull plates is theoretically purported to relieve pressure on the Dura Mater along the spinal column that can produce pain when injured or agitated. The Dura Mater is the protective sheath that covers the brain and spinal cord and is attached to the brain at the top of the spine and to the great nerve trunks as they leave the spinal cord and travel out into the body. An injury such as whiplash or Atlas subluxation could seriously aggravate this area, causing pain.

4) Bowen Therapy — Bowen therapy is a technique of soft tissue release developed in Australia in the 1950's. Its goal is to reset the autonomic nervous system and stimulate the body to heal itself. This gentle therapy is a unique form of neuromuscular re-patterning, working primarily on the nervous system on a structural and energetic level. Structurally, the method of treatment uses a series of gentle rolling moves done in sets on the connective tissues with resting pauses in between each set. These pauses allow the body time to process the treatment and benefit from each set of moves.

The practitioner is responsible for choosing the appropriate combinations of sequences of moves they feel will address the body as a whole or target a more specific problem. The practitioner also aims to remove any stress build up found in the body during the treatment. Energetically, this therapy aims to achieve a level of relaxation in the body that stimulates energy flow and homeostasis on a cellular level, which allows the body to begin its own healing and restorative processes. Aside from restoring the body's energetic balance and healing ability, Bowen therapy is also successful in relieving pain in a wide variety of musculoskeletal and internal conditions, including chronic FMS.

5) Breathing Exercises — The stress of chronic FMS can cause poor breathing habits to develop, such as shallow breathing into the chest cavity due to pain, weakness, or muscle tension. Practicing deep breathing from the abdomen helps you get sufficient oxygen delivered through the lungs into the bloodstream and to all the cells in the body. These cells require sufficient oxygen for cellular respiration and cell metabolism. Shallow breathing inhibits the body from expelling sufficient levels of carbon dioxide, which is very unhealthy. Practicing deep breathing from the abdomen increases lung capacity, increases energy production, relieves anxiety, lowers stress levels and blood pressure, improves brain function, and can relieve asthma symptoms and insomnia.

It is good to practice deep breathing at least every morning and evening, but should be done during the day whenever needed. Practicing deep breathing is simple: For five minutes, three times a day, slowly breathe in through your nose expanding the diaphragm, the strongest muscle in the abdomen, until the lungs are comfortably full. Hold the breath for up to ten seconds. Place the tongue between the roof of your mouth and your front teeth, allow your lower jaw to hang loosely, and exhale slowly through the mouth. To relax quickly, stretch the arms upward and out in a "V" shape above your head during inhalation and bring them down to your sides during exhalation. This can help with anxiety attacks under high stress situations and can be repeated as needed.

6) Chiropractic Spinal Manipulation — Chiropractors are licensed doctors (DC) in all 50 states in the U.S. and are the third largest group of health care providers in our nation, after medical doctors and dentists. They are recognized by the U.S. Department of Health and Human Resources as providing "proven treatment" for a variety of conditions and are the most widely used practitioners in the alternative health care field. Most health care insurance plans cover chiropractic visits up to a set maximum per year or per condition and many will go beyond the policy maximum if the treatment plan is proven to be medically necessary.

Chiropractic treatment is based on the belief the health of the body can be greatly compromised when a spinal subluxation occurs (a vertebra that is not moving properly or is out of alignment). When a subluxation of the spine occurs, the normal flow of impulses to and from the brain are disrupted or distorted, and are not able to travel freely along the spinal cord to and from the various organs and soft tissues of the body. This can result in inflammation and pain in nerves, muscles, tendons, ligaments, bones, and joints, as well as other physical disorders.

Chiropractic manipulation of the spine aims to correct any spinal subluxations and restore the central nervous system to normal functioning. This, in turn, restores the body's ability to heal itself. Chiropractic treatment is well known for its success in relieving back pain and muscle spasms and is also used to treat arthritis, bursitis, sinusitis, migraines, and other headaches. It is a natural therapy, using a variety of non-invasive techniques, and does not involve the use of drugs or surgery.

7) Feldendrais Method — The Feldenkrais Method of Somatic Education is a method of movement developed by Moshe Feldenkrais in the 1940's and is based on the brain's innate capacity for learning and its potential for lifelong development and growth. The benefits of the Feldenkrais method range from reducing pain, improving neurologically based difficulties and learning disabilities, to increasing mobility. Its original purpose was to enhance the performance of professional dancers, musicians, actors, and athletes.

The Feldenkrais Method is taught in two modalities: 1) Awareness Through Movement (ATM) and 2) Functional Integration. Certified practitioners who teach these modalities to "students" all receive training that is approved and regulated by the Feldenkrais Guild of North America's Training Board. ATM is taught in group sessions where the practitioner leads the students through a series of structured movement sequences designed to establish new patterns of movement, evoking a more synergistic use of oneself and the ability to move with more comfort, ease, and inner authority.

Functional Integration is taught one on one in a hands-on interaction with the practitioner through slow, gentle, non-invasive touch. The student is guided through a series of precise movements that relax tense areas, alter habitual patterns of tension, and provide new information to the neuromuscular system. The Feldenkrais Method shows how to learn from your body, gives you an effective means to take charge of your own care, and provides results almost immediately. It differs from massage in that it attempts to alter the body's structure to provide more lasting and even life-long benefits.

The goal of the Feldenkrais Method is to teach you to move with minimum effort and maximum efficiency and flexibility by aligning you with gravity, increasing your kinesthetic senses, and becoming more aware of how your body works. Integrating movement with thinking, feeling, and sensing improves posture and breathing, reduces stress, tension, and fatigue, and eases pain and stiffness. Students learn dynamic balance using natural gravity, not muscular strength, and learn to move with grace, ease, and elegance.

When you are aligned with gravity, you feel a sense of lightness and ease that allows the body and the nervous system to adapt to changing conditions. This also allows you to use a variety of movements that prevent "static load" (energy congestion) to develop in muscles that can result in stiffness, strain, and painful injury to connective tissues. Ultimately, the student acquires a means of gaining a degree of control over their pain, finds more comfortable positions for their body to move in throughout the day, and learns to experience more frequently the organic pleasure that comes from ordinary movements.

8) Heat & Cold Therapy — The use of heat therapy is an immediate and convenient tool to help relieve aches and pains in your own home. Applying heat to selected areas of pain increases the circulation to the area, helps muscle groups relax, reduces stiffness and "knots" in the muscles, and increases mobility. Moist heat is the best kind of heat to apply to an area of pain. Delivered via a warm shower or a wet towel heated under hot tap water, moist heat is able to get to hard to reach places that other therapies may have a difficult time accessing. This is also one of the easiest, least disruptive courses of therapy available.

Because the towel will only hold the heat for a relatively short time, the danger of too much heat exposure is eliminated, as in the case of a heating pad that is often left on much too long. The rule of thumb is twenty minutes on/ twenty minutes off. Unless you have phlebitis, other vascular problems, or a recent injury, it is often helpful to massage the area after you remove the moist heat to help dissipate the heat and further relax the area. Back, neck, and shoulder pain responds well to moist heat therapy.

The use of cold therapy is a way to reduce pain from swelling and is often used to treat muscle strain, sprain, and other injuries. In such cases, cold packs applied to the area of pain should be used alone for no longer than twenty minutes at a time and no more than the first twenty-four to thirty-six hours. Cold can be easily applied by using a frozen gel pack, an ice pack, or a bag of frozen peas. A cold pack massage can also be helpful by rubbing the area of pain in a circular motion with the cold pack for five to seven minutes. Lower back pain is particularly responsive to ice rubs. Be sure to wrap the cold pack in a towel before you apply it to the skin to avoid ice-burn.

Alternating the use of hot and cold therapy can sometimes be the best way to treat pain and soreness, such as a painful, stiff neck. First, take a hot shower to relax, followed by a five to seven minute ice massage to further relieve pain and inflammation. The rule in finding the right treatment for your problem is to experiment, first by trying one method of treatment a few times and, if it does not seem to be helping, try the other a few times.

Then, if you are still not getting relief, try alternating hot and cold treatments until you find the best way to relieve your discomfort. If the pain persists and you are not sure of its cause, consult your health care provider. I have found that an oblong icepack wrapped in a thin kitchen towel wrapped around the back of my neck for up to twenty minutes or so does wonders for FMS pain and calms down and dulls the pain signals from the body to the brain via the neck. This also helps ease headache pain as well.

9) Magnet Therapy — The use of magnet therapy became popular in the U.S. after having been used in Europe and the Far East for some time and is used primarily to relieve pain and promote healing. Research in the U.S. on the effectiveness of magnet therapy has shown that magnets sewn into socks alleviate the chronic pain of diabetic peripheral neuropathy (chronic pain caused by nerve deterioration in the feet). Also, double-blind studies have demonstrated that magnetic stimulation of the brain can ease severe depression, and magnets can provide relief for painful post-polio syndrome.

Magnets work on the theory that, by increasing circulation and blood flow to an affected area, swelling and inflammation are reduced and pain is alleviated. This is accomplished by applying a magnet of a negative (north field) designation to the affected area with a gauss range of 400-2,500. A refrigerator magnet, for instance, is about 200 gauss. Magnets of a positive (south field) designation do not work.

Magnets are available in a variety of forms and can be used on a variety of disorders. They are sold as kneepads, chair pads, bracelets, wraps for the neck, back or other parts of the body, and as mattress pads. Besides helping diabetic neuropathy and severe depression, other conditions helped by magnet therapy are: arthritis; asthma; carpal tunnel syndrome; chronic fibromyalgia; infections; migraines; osteoporosis; ruptured disks; sports injuries; and tennis elbow.

You should never use magnets if you are pregnant, use an insulin pump, an automatic defibrillator, or have a pacemaker. Always check with your doctor before trying magnet therapy to be sure it is safe for you and only use magnets that are designated for use on the human body.

10) Massage Therapy — The hands-on therapy of massage entails the manipulation of soft tissues such as muscles, tendons, and ligaments. Massage has been an effective healing therapy for centuries and is well known throughout many cultures in the world. Massage works to relieve pain and discomfort and promote healing in a variety of ways: by promoting muscle relaxation; stimulating blood flow into the soft tissues; reducing inflammation by increasing lymphatic circulation; breaking up scar tissue and adhesions; promoting drainage of the sinus fluids; and improving sleep.

It can be an effective therapy for a number of conditions, such as: arthritis; asthma; depression; diabetes; headaches; insomnia; muscle pain; spasms; and stress. In addition, in 1999 the American Massage Therapy Association stated that a study done by the Touch Research Institute at the University of Miami on women with breast cancer showed that massage therapy done three times a week for five weeks showed an 80% improvement in immune functions.

There are many forms of massage that involve varying techniques and pressures. Deep muscle massage performed with strong pressure should be avoided by anyone with a history of phlebitis, high blood pressure, or any other vascular disorder. No form of massage should be performed on inflamed areas or on anyone with an infectious or malignant condition. Check with your doctor to see if you are a safe candidate for massage therapy before you try it. The various forms of massage currently in use are based on different theories and utilize different specific techniques. For example, deep tissue massage which focuses on releasing chronic muscle tension in specific problem areas, is applied with greater pressure and on deeper muscles than Swedish massage.

To name a few, I will begin with *Cranial Massage*. Like *bio-cranial therapy*, cranial massage aims at gently relaxing and releasing tissues surrounding the cranium that have become chronically tight. This tension pulls on the back of the neck, which in turn tugs on the ligaments at the base of the brain connected to the foramen magnum and the pain sensitive Dura. These tiny ligaments attach inside the base of the skull and tug on the tissues that transmit pain signals to the brain, causing migraine headaches and body-wide pain. Releasing this tension can relieve headaches and body pain for periods of time that can last from a couple of days to a couple of months.

Neuromuscular Massage concentrates on using finger pressure on sensitive "trigger points" to release energy congestion and increase blood flow and is another form of deep tissue massage. *Reflexology* is a very old massage method originating in China and has been popular in the U.S. since the 1950's. It applies pressure to different spots on the feet, hands, and ears that are believed to correlate with specific areas and organs in the body. Its aim is to open channels for energy flow to affected areas of the body to relieve pain and promote healing. This can be a method of treating yourself by learning the pressure points that are effective for relieving pain.

Rolfing, or *Structural Integration,* is a method of deep massage used to align the body, restore balance, and improve mobility by manipulating the connective tissues linking muscles to bones. The therapist achieves this by releasing deeply held stress through the use of fingertips, knuckles, elbows, and knees to apply intense pressure to tendons and ligaments. The result can increase overall range of motion and decrease body pain. This method does not promote relaxation during its application and can be very painful.

Shiatsu Massage is the oriental massage from Japan that means "finger pressure" and focuses on acupressure points to restore and maintain health. The shiatsu therapist unblocks congested energy by applying firm, rhythmic pressure to specific points along the meridians of the body for three to ten seconds each. Unblocking the energy at key pressure points allows it to flow freely through the meridians in the body, promoting healing and relieving pain.

Sports Massage is a method of combining kneading, passive stretching and a range of deep tissue motion designed to increase flexibility and ease muscle strain after exercising.

Swedish Massage is a specific technique developed in the early 1800's by Peter Hendricks Ling to induce the body to relax and promote rehabilitation after an injury by reducing swelling and soreness. The method uses a combination of kneading, stroking, tapping, and shaking and is less intense than deep tissue massage.

Remember, it is always a good idea to check with your doctor about a massage method that appeals to you before you try it and make sure it is safe and fits your particular needs. If you suffer from fibromyalgia, do not allow any massage therapist to do deep massage on your muscles and do not allow anyone to ever massage the neck.

11) Meditation — Meditation is a self-care technique used as an effective means of reducing the anxiety and tension that contribute to the intensity and duration of chronic pain. Meditation has been practiced for thousands of years and aims to relax the body and calm the mind by keeping it focused on the present.

Most meditation techniques fall into two categories: concentrative and mindfulness.

Concentrative meditation calms the mind by focusing the attention on a single sound, object, or the breath. The most common method is focusing on the breath while sitting or lying in comfortable and quiet environment. By closing the eyes and inhaling through the nose for three seconds and exhaling through the mouth for five, you can develop a slow, deep, regular rhythm to the breath that allows your mind to become tranquil and aware. After ten to twenty minutes of meditation, the mind and body can feel the benefits of having taken a refreshing nap.

Mindful meditation allows the mind to become aware of the variety of feelings, thoughts, and sensations of its current reality without reacting to them. This method attains a calm state in the mind by sitting quietly and allowing the images of your surroundings to pass through the mind without becoming attached to them in any way, or becoming involved with them through any kind of reaction. It is a very disciplined practice with the same benefits as concentrative meditation.

Transcendental Meditation (TM) is another form of *concentrative* meditation that brings about a state of deep relaxation in the body while the mind is highly alert. There have been vast studies done on TM that show its effectiveness in controlling anxiety, reducing stress, reducing high blood pressure, enhancing the immune system, controlling substance abuse, and treating chronic pain. The TM method involves being assigned a specific sound by a trained practitioner that he or she feels matches your overall persona. You then sit in a quite place, close your eyes, and, after voicing the sound out loud a few times, begin repeating it silently and gently in your mind in a rhythmic loop to your own liking, allowing your thoughts to pass through the mind freely without reacting to them. After a twenty-minute meditation the benefits are said to be equal to a refreshing night's sleep: a clear, alert mind and relaxed and energized body.

12) Osteopathic Manipulation Therapy — Osteopathy or osteopathic manipulation therapy (OMT) is a hands-on therapy developed in the U.S. in 1874 and is currently performed by a licensed osteopath (DO). A doctor of osteopathy is licensed as such after completing special training in addition to regular medical school, and has the same skills as a fully trained medical doctor. In addition to performing OMT, a doctor of osteopathy can diagnose conditions, prescribe drugs, perform surgery, order tests, admit and discharge patients, and treat in all the same ways as a regular medical doctor.

DOs often specialize in family medicine and make wonderful family physicians. An osteopath is specially trained in the highly skilled method of light touch called palpation and uses this skill to locate and assess any maladies in the musculoskeletal system. Combining palpation with regular medical methods, the osteopath can diagnose a problem, devise an appropriate treatment plan, and usually has an overall understanding and respect for alternative therapies.

When OMT is indicated as beneficial, the patient is given a series of treatments where they lie down on a table and are usually asked to first change into a light robe over the torso. OMT involves a variety of gentle release techniques focusing on soft tissues, bones, and joints. It aims to improve overall mobility, increase range of motion, and provide relief from pain. This treatment focuses on facilitating alignment and mobility of the spinal column to eliminate any pressure or obstruction to nerves and arteries that result in a wide variety of physical malfunctions and disorders. OMT is also used to balance energy through pressure points along acupuncture meridians to release the flow of blocked or congested (static) energy. It is a non-invasive therapy that promotes healing and is helpful in relieving chronic muscle pain and tension.

13) Non-Surgical Spinal Decompression Therapy — This gentle and non-invasive therapy is offered without drugs, injections, or surgery through a new state of the art machine called the DRX-9000. This spinal decompression machine treats back pain and sciatica caused by: bulging or herniated discs; degenerative disc disease; facet syndrome; and failed back surgery. It is an easy and comfortable way to decompress (relieve pressure) between vertebrae that have been affected by trauma or illness.

The machine does this by pulling the spine in two directions at once, creating a slight suction and more space between each vertebra. This allows oozing disc gel to return to the center of disc in the case of bulging or herniated discs, sucks the disc back into the space between the vertebrae, and also takes pressure off the nerves that cause sciatica. Bernard Zeliger, DO, Founding Dean of Touro University College of Osteopathic Medicine, Vallejo, CA said about this therapy, "As a surgeon, I only want to do surgery when I absolutely have to. Non-Surgical Spinal Decompression Therapy gives my patients a more conservative treatment option that can eliminate the need for surgery altogether, and that's a very good thing!"

14) Transcutaneous Electrical Nerve Stimulation Therapy (Tens) — Tens unit therapy is a micro-current therapy that aims at relieving pain and controlling muscle spasms, increasing the rate of healing for injuries and fractures, and is believed to stimulate the production of the body's natural painkillers: endorphins. In addition, researchers state micro-current therapy increases the concentration in the body of ATP (the

body's bio-chemical energy) up to five times normal levels. Tens therapy first appeared in scientific literature in 1975 and is now commonly available in doctor's offices and physiotherapy clinics.

It can also be performed at home by purchasing a battery powered mobile Tens unit. Electrodes are strategically placed on the skin and joined to the Tens unit with wires delivering a low voltage electrical signal to nerve endings, blocking pain signals before they reach the brain. The theory behind this is, by electrically stimulating the nerves in an affected area, normal pain signals become scrambled and ineffective. Tens therapy is said to be safe and have no known side effects and therefore can theoretically be used as often as necessary. Relief from chronic pain and muscle spasms can be short-term or long-term.

Exercise Therapies

Research has shown that exercise is key to managing chronic pain. However, with FMS, chronic pain can be exacerbated with some forms of exercise that are too strenuous for soft tissues in this condition, and a very conservative approach to exercise must be taken. Soft tissues that are chronically constricted and fatigued need to be very gently stretched so circulation is increased to feed and cleanse what have become toxic, nutrition-deprived tissues.

In addition, tissues that have become weakened or atrophied from lack of use need to be very carefully lengthened, strengthened, and brought back into a state of mobility and tone. When the pain of FMS prohibits the kind of exercise that raises the heart rate, works the muscle groups, and causes perspiration, such as aerobic exercises and lifting weights, other forms of exercise need to be used in their place. When you exert muscles that are already chronically tight, due to a resting potential that is set too high from distorted nerve impulses coming from the brain into soft tissues, they become strained and injured and the pain can be dramatically exacerbated.

When you do not move the muscles at all to avoid pain, they begin to atrophy, and the downward spiral of ever increasing weakness, fatigue, chronic pain, and depression is inevitable. The only way to avoid this is to keep moving your body in safe ways that will not cause injury to the soft tissues or drastically exacerbate symptoms. It is also vital to get lots of rest, eat right, and take the appropriate nutritional supplements to help in building and repairing the muscles.

1) Warm Water Pool Physical Therapy — If you have been bed-ridden, house bound, or unable to walk further than the next room due to chronic

pain, warm water pool therapy is a wonderful way to begin moving your body. Facilities that provide this type of exercise usually require an order from your doctor and will put you on a waiting list if classes are full. Classes are usually offered at various times throughout the day and are taught by an instructor licensed in warm water rehabilitation therapy. The warm water, about ninety-two degrees, gently relaxes your muscles and calms down pain signals by disrupting and/or distracting them with the pleasing and soothing sensations that come from the water and the support the water gives the body.

The movements in warm water pool rehabilitation therapy are designed to be gentle, easy, and appropriate for all kinds of conditions, such as chronic pain disorders, arthritis, heart disease, joint replacements, spinal reconstruction, musculoskeletal disorders, and other neurological disorders. The water supports the weight of the body and limbs so that deconditioned muscles are not likely to become strained. The repetitions of each exercise are kept to a minimum of around eight reps per set and a routine of exercises usually lasts about 45 minutes. The facilities provide clean hot showers and dressing rooms, and a nice hot shower after a work out can be very relaxing and beneficial.

When you return home, it is always a good idea to lie down and rest or, even better, to take a nap so the muscles can process the work out and recover from the movements and stretches. When you wake, always rise very slowly, beginning with rolling over on your side and then gently and slowly lifting your legs off the edge of the bed while pushing yourself up to a sit position. Rising by sitting up in bed or rising too quickly will startle the CNS and cause agitation to the system.

Also, always remember to stand up slowly, stretch upward from the back of the spine, and go calmly on your way. It is a good idea to drink a large glass of water right after each class or exercise to flush out toxins released into the bloodstream from the soft tissues through the increase in blood flow that results from exercising. Attending a warm water exercise class on a twice per week basis with a couple days in between is a safe way to begin.

After your body gets used to exercising twice a week without experiencing brief soft tissue pain flare-ups, and you are feeling noticeably stronger, increase to a maximum of three times a week. Over time, your body will gain strength and mobility, more efficient circulation, increased energy, and your pain levels will come down. You may experience a brief increase in pain levels shortly after you get out of the water, so be very careful not to over-do it while the pain levels are lowered in the warm, soothing water.

Take it slow and easy and stick with it. It will not be long before you see an improvement in your overall condition. Once you have become stronger and feel you are ready to take your exercise out of the water, the next step is choosing a gentle form of exercise on land. Walking is always a great form of gentle exercise. Another form is gentle Thai Chi.

2) Tai Chi - Gentle — Tai Chi is a moving meditation that originated in ancient China. It has been practiced for centuries throughout the world and is suitable for almost everyone. Tai Chi is a slow, gentle series of beautiful, deliberate movements designed to integrate the body and mind in ways that improves overall health and mental alertness. The benefits of Tai Chi are many and include: improving muscular strength, flexibility, and stamina; improving relaxation, balance, and posture; and improving circulation and immunity. As a result of increasing flexibility and strength of muscles that support and protect the joints, pain and stiffness can be greatly reduced.

Tai Chi is also beneficial in reducing and managing stress and relieving the pain of arthritis and many other painful musculoskeletal conditions. Tai Chi aims to bring tranquility to the mind, which is the basis for concentration and alertness. It also aims to gather the Chi, or life force energy, and open up the energy gates of the body so the Chi can strengthen as it flows along the meridians. Tai Chi also aims to unify the strength of the body and develop the Chi into spiritual awareness and enlightenment (being attuned to the now). The result is a body that is strong, relaxed, agile, graceful, and peaceful.

My Tai Chi instructor, Lydia Olson, wrote about how Tai Chi works, "Tai Chi is an internal art. It involves the mind, the inside body and the inner power – the Chi. It gathers the Chi to penetrate the pathways. The Chi moves the blood and the blood moves the nutrients to give supply to what your body needs. Blood also moves the toxins out of your body so when the energy gates open, your chi gets in more effectively. Tai Chi exercise will decrease feelings of stress, and improve concentration, posture, balance, circulation and overall health."

The Chinese consider Tai Chi to be an integral part of their traditional medicine practice. This form of exercise is commonly learned in a classroom setting and can also be done at home, guided by recorded visual instruction. It involves being on your feet for about forty-five minutes, so you need to be sure that you have enough stamina to support yourself for that long. Begin with one class per week and increase from there.

3) Qi Gong - Gentle — Qi Gong (pronounced chie-goong) is an ancient form of Chinese exercise that is older than Tai Chi. "Qi" means life force

energy and "Gong" means a skilled practice of work. Qi Gong is a slow motion exercise concentrating on combining breathing meditation and movement to increase emotional and physical health and the vital life force energy of the entire body. It should be taught by a trained professional, can be quickly learned, and is easily practiced in your own home.

The discipline of Qi Gong aims to improve your mental clarity, strengthen the muscles and joints, and improve balance. According to traditional Chinese medicine, the practice of Qi Gong is effective in preventing illness by increasing levels of endorphins, the body's natural biochemical painkillers, that relieve pain and help maintain mental health.

By combining the exercises with proper breathing, the physical and mental processes operate in balance to promote healing, relaxation, and increased internal energy. Qi Gong can be effective in reducing blood pressure, reducing stress and anxiety, and alleviating pain and depression. Qi Gong is not strenuous and is very good for beginners or people who suffer from chronic pain.

4) Pilates - Modified — Pilates is a very popular modality of exercising for a wide variety of objectives, whether it be to improve performance in areas such as sports or dancing or help people recover more quickly from soft tissue injuries. Pilates can also be helpful with other physical problems, such as chronic fatigue, back pain, and arthritis, or it can simply be used to improve overall health and fitness. Pilates was originally developed by Joseph H. Pilates and brought by him to the U.S. in the 1920's.

Pilates is taught one on one or in a class setting, and the client is given a specific program to fit their particular needs. Today in the U.S., Pilates has been re-configured by a popular Hollywood fitness instructor by the name of Mari Winsor, who has reorganized Pilates to benefit a wide range of objectives. She began as a personal fitness trainer and has branched out into providing instructional DVDs under the name of "Winsor Pilates," where she becomes your personal trainer and shows you the exercises by using several model students.

Winsor Pilates provides many individual programs, including sculpting workouts for the abs, back, upper body, buns, and thighs, an accelerated body sculpting workout, and a 20-minute basic workout. Her method provides a modified version of each exercise for people with back or neck issues and these modified versions are suitable to those with FMS. You will need a good one and a half inch thick workout mat for your floor, for a few minutes a day.

This method requires the ability to exercise on land against gravity and should be tried cautiously, using the modified exercises only. As with each modality of exercise, check with your doctor first to make sure it is safe for you in your current physical state. The aim of Pilates is to release stress, improve balance and strength, and increase overall health and flexibility in the mind and body.

5) Yoga - Restorative — Yoga has been around for over 5,000 years, originated in India, and is used world wide to unite the mind, body, and spirit. It teaches you to still a restless and noisy mind while exercising the body. The term Hatha is a Sandskrit word that means "willful" and the term yoga means "union." Although Hatha Yoga is a familiar term to those who practice yoga, it does not represent any particular style, although its postures are practiced with an emphasis on breath, stability, and mobility to facilitate mind-body balance. There are many different styles of yoga and some are soft and easy while others are strenuous and difficult to do. For the FMS patient, it would be wise to only use a gentle style of yoga to begin with and beginners should start with an easy style.

A Few Styles of Yoga:

- *Ananda yoga* is a slower-paced style, cultivates spirituality by teaching meditation, and appeals to beginners.
- *Ashtanga yoga* uses postures linked together in a continuous flow and performed while practicing "ujjayi" (oo-ja-yee) breathing, a style of breathing exclusive to yoga. Ashtanga yoga, or power yoga, begins easy and becomes more strenuous as the student progresses, building stamina, strength, and flexibility. This style is not for beginners.
- *Bikram yoga* is a sequential series of twenty-six postures practiced in a continuous flow and, because it requires a great deal of work, it is also not for beginners. This style of yoga is practiced in a room heated at 100 degrees or more to promote sweating to cleanse the body of toxins.
- *Kundalini and Tantra yoga* both focus on activating the chakras, the seven energy centers or core of the body. This style of yoga sees the body as a river of energy and explores moving the center of the body and not the limbs.
- *Raja* is good for beginners because it focuses more on meditation and on spiritual strength.
- *Sevananda yoga* focuses on five basic principles that unite the body, mind (intellect), the spirit, and the heart. These principles take a holistic approach to health and include pranayama (proper breathing), savasana (proper relaxation), meditation, a vegetarian diet, and the study of the Vedic scriptures. This is also very good for beginners.

- *Tivamukti yoga* is a style of yoga taught in a classroom setting and focuses on spiritual teaching, readings, chanting, meditation, and postures. This form is good for beginners, too.
- *Yin* yoga is a quiet and deeply reflective practice utilizing long held poses (three to five minutes) for the purpose of stimulating the "chi health flow" along the meridians of the body. Like all yoga, it strengthens connective tissue and joints and encourages psychological wellbeing.

Other styles of yoga include: *Kripalu* yoga that focuses on integrating breath, movement, and body alignment; *Integral* yoga, *Phoenix Rising* yoga, and *Lyengar* yoga, which all focus on gentle postures that are very good for beginners or for people who are out of shape. Each yoga style is taught by a qualified teacher and has a variety of unique techniques and methods; however, the goals remain the same.

The goals are to: remove blocks from the body to allow a freer flow of energy; enhance well-being; achieve inner peace; acquire a greater understanding and awareness of the mind/body/spirit connection; free the self from negative thinking patterns that deplete the body of its vital energies; increase strength, flexibility, and mobility; and ultimately bring balance to the mind, body, and spirit as one whole living system.

Yoga can bring relief to a wide variety of physical conditions. As always, check with your doctor to make sure the style of yoga that appeals to you is safe for you to try at the present time. If you join a one-hour class, try using the restful position of "child's pose" when a pose seems too intense or between the poses you cannot do at first. When you sign up, be sure your new yoga class is under the category of "restorative yoga."

Psychotherapies

The primary goal of psychotherapy (talk-therapy) is to create and/or restore mental health and balance and to eliminate possible ill effects caused by depression or psychological distress. This can be achieved through the use of a number of methods, either by themselves or in combination with each other, that heal emotional, psychological, and spiritual wounds. Through psychotherapy you can learn to better understand your condition, identify and change unhealthy thoughts and behaviors, set realistic life goals, and find better ways to cope with and solve problems. It also teaches healthy guidelines pertaining to behavior towards others.

Healthy guidelines include: the skill of self-control through internal and external boundary setting; respecting the boundaries of others; concentrating on your own life and not the lives of others; and respecting the human rights and freedoms of others to live their lives as they see fit without judging. Judging others includes: disagreeing with the way they chose to live (a negative value judgment); seeing another person as being "less than" in some way; or assigning negative labels and names to someone.

Assessing another person for health, safety, and appropriateness is not judging. It is basic self-care that assesses and recognizes the behaviors of others and acknowledges whether or not it is healthy or safe to have contact with them.

Psychotherapy can be short-term or it can involve many sessions over several years. There are also numerous methods of therapy available. Some focus on understanding past issues while others focus on the present and changing current unhealthy, counter-productive behaviors.

These therapies include: behavior therapy; cognitive therapy; dialectic behavioral therapy; eye movement desensitization & reprocessing (EMDR); emotional freedom technique therapy; existential therapy; family/marital therapy; Gestalt therapy; humanistic therapy; interpersonal therapy; neuro-linguistic programming (NLP); psychoanalytic therapy; rational emotive behavior therapy (REBT); reality therapy; thought field therapy; transactional analysis; transference-focused psychotherapy (TFP); and transpersonal psychotherapy, to name a few.

Depending on the severity of the patient's depression, both individual and group therapy modalities can be used. Many therapists combine talk therapy and homework assignments of specific reading between sessions. This can speed up the process and make the most efficient use of this expensive treatment.

The sixteenth century alchemist Paracelsus believed that all painful emotions are brought about "when a person's intellect has been unable to cope with that which has presented itself for his cognition." He goes on to say, "The more the soul learns concerning the being and the aim of the human spirit, the less the soul will need to appeal to the services of the Alchemist, for then will the soul – recognizing and acknowledging the why and the wherefore of all things – be able and ready alone to cope with everything that may come its way. It will know how to adjust itself to all the situations of life and will derive its joys and its happiness from a wealth of capabilities – from an initiative power for creating new possibilities, even when it seems as though life were spent and threatened to lose its way amid the quick sands. Ripe souls, such as these, are no longer slaves – they are the masters of their perceptions. The rising mist of uncontrollable emotions no longer dims the Windows of the Soul, for – having learnt to regard its own being objectively – it has weaned itself from tears. Such a soul will then have attained so far upon the Path of Learning as to have ridded itself of the pressure of false presentiments concerning the World."

To my knowledge, a better argument for engaging in the learning process of psychotherapy could be not written. In these few words, Paracelsus so eloquently explains all of the solid benefits of becoming an expert on your self, your life, your mind, and your condition. Learning to understand yourself and your past lays the foundation for the strength and confidence necessary to allow you to genuinely heal and release useless and painfully negative memories, while at the same time choosing to retain the useful, happy, and positive ones.

We are all meant to grow, learn, and change; a failure to do so is unnatural and unhealthy. The choice to become an enlightened being is simply that: a choice. Everyone has to start somewhere and it may take you a few years of learning before you get a handle on your self and your life, but you are going to be a few years older anyway. Do you really want to be stuck in the same place you are now in five years, living a stagnant life, thinking stagnant thoughts, or would you rather see where you can lead yourself, how rich your life can be, and what possibilities await you?

No matter what your challenges are, there is always a way to grow personally, evolve spiritually, improve your life, and keep yourself continuously moving forward. It just takes beginning somewhere. Getting an idea about the kinds of help that are available to choose from can be very helpful and this section will go into some of those choices. I will discuss a few therapies I feel might be particularly helpful to people who are suffering from chronic fibromyalgia. These methods are highly effective in alleviating chronic pain and depression and can be very helpful in integrating both the mind and body with a state of increased health and wellbeing.

1) Behavioral Therapy — This type of therapy uses a system of rewarding and reinforcing positive behavior. This includes the process of desensitization that involves confronting whatever is causing fear, anxiety, and discomfort and overcoming those responses. This form of therapy focuses on your current problems, stays away from past experiences, and can be used in combination with other therapies.

2) Cognitive Therapy — This type of therapy is based on the premise that how you view your current life is determined by your past experiences.

Although past experiences are therefore an important part of this thera-peutic process, cognitive therapy focuses on your current problems and changing any self-defeating or self-destructive feelings and behaviors. It does this by helping the patient identify the distorted thought (cognitive) patterns causing them to view and interpret their current reality through the lens of their dead past. This type of therapy also helps teach mental discipline.

3) Cognitive-Behavioral Therapy — This type of therapy is based on the premise that the patient's thoughts, and not life situations or other people, determine their behavior. It combines cognitive and behavioral therapy techniques and works with the past and present to identify unhealthy, negative, inappropriate beliefs and behaviors and replaces them with healthy, positive, appropriate ones.

4) Dialectical-Behavioral Therapy (DBT) — This type of therapy was originally designed for patients who suffer from Borderline Personality Disorder who exhibit suicidal behavior, but has been adapted for people with other serious psychological conditions as well. DBT is a form of cognitive-behavioral therapy focusing on teaching patients behavioral skills to better tolerate stress, regulate their emotions, and improve their relationships by helping them to better understand healthy boundaries and appropriate ways to interact with others.

5) Interpersonal Therapy — This type of therapy teaches patients how to evaluate the way they interact with others and focuses on their current relationships with others. The goal of this therapy is to improve interper-sonal skills and develop healthy strategies for dealing with problems in both relationships and communication. This therapy can be used for many types of behavioral challenges; however, treating the behaviors of patients suffering from psychological personality disorders such as Bor-derline Personality Disorder and Narcissistic Personality Disorders are only likely to improve marginally.

6) Psychoanalysis — This type of therapy is based on the theory that the unconscious mind determines how you think, feel, and behave and is cre-ated by childhood events and biological urges. Psychoanalysis evolved out of the theories of Dr. Sigmund Freud and is an intensive, long-term therapy often involving a few sessions a week for several years. It is now considered an outdated approach.

Psychoanalysis focuses on examining memories, events, and feelings from the past for the purpose of understanding the unconscious motivations for current feelings and behaviors. It aims to make changes to improve the patient's life by talking about and exploring whatever comes to mind. During therapy, the patient usually lies on a couch while the therapist sits in a chair behind them and takes notes.

7) Psychodynamic Psychotherapy — This type of therapy is based on the theories of psychoanalysis, however it is less intense, less frequent (usually once a week), and involves a shorter time period (usually less than one year). It has become one of the most common modalities of therapy and focuses on increasing awareness of unconscious thoughts and behaviors. By the patient developing new insights into their unconscious motivations, they can use this new awareness to acknowledge the link between thoughts, feelings, and behaviors (their symptoms) and their unconscious meaning or motivation.

With this new understanding they can modify unwanted behaviors and thoughts and are better able to resolve conflicts and live happier lives. Unlike psychotherapy, the patient and therapist sit face to face. This form of therapy is likely to show benefits to people suffering with emotional illness and may not be as affective for people suffering from serious psychological disorders.

8) Transference-Focused Psychotherapy (TFP) — This type of therapy is an intensive talk therapy originally designed to reduce symptoms and improve functionality in patients with Borderline Personality Disorder. In 2007, TFP was tested in a randomized study done by John F. Clarkson, Ph.D. from Weill Medical College at Cornell University in New York City and was shown to improve symptoms of depression, anxiety, and suicidal thoughts.

Learning how to reduce the stressors in your life that are not easy to eliminate, such as the stress caused by chronic FMS, is vitally important to healing and includes developing the ability to monitor and control the thoughts you are choosing to think while you are thinking them. This is especially difficult when your brain is being bombarded with pain signals, is chronically fatigued, and in a state of fibro-fog.

However, it is absolutely necessary to acquire this skill so you can avoid bathing your body in the deadly stress hormones of adrenaline and cortisol released by negative thoughts, fears, and their subsequent emotions. Stress hormones can exacerbate any condition, especially those conditions based in the central nervous system, such as FMS.

Learning how to choose your thoughts wisely and use your mind as a helpful tool requires fully realizing that you are not your mind, nor are you a ganglion mass of habitual thought patterns. The human brain is simply another biological organ located inside the skull performing a great many functions, and only one of them happens to be thinking. You are not your thoughts; you are consciousness, and can purposefully become the observer of your thoughts and behaviors. You, as the conscious observer, can become the master of your own mind and learn to pick and choose the very thoughts you think that determine your responses, your emotions, your behaviors, and the direction you will take in healing your chronic FMS.

You can choose to think thoughts that are informed, correct, appropriate, and healthy and choose to discard or ignore thoughts that are not. Repetitive thoughts create and energetically feed and deepen their own pathways in the brain, and will become habitual. Conversely, when you stop feeding energy to repetitive thoughts by choosing not to think them, their pathways energetically starve, shrink, and eventually let go of the thoughts or thought patterns altogether.

This phenomenon is very much like a story I like to tell about an old Himalayan monk who habitually traveled the same pathway every day to the temple on top of the mountain. Day after day the monk walked up and down the same side of the same mountain. The more the monk walked upon the path, the deeper, more permanent, and more easily accessible the pathway became. It became so easy and habitual he soon was able to traverse the path without being aware that he was doing so. He just went up the mountain automatically, turning at each switch back with the same ease as the day before.

One day, out of curiosity, the monk decided to choose a different path up the other side of the mountain. This took some daily effort on his part and was not easy at first, and he had to pay close attention to where he was going, but the monk did not consider the difficulty of the change. He simply committed himself to the new path as he had always done with every path he had ever chosen throughout his life.

Soon the new path became unexpectedly enjoyable to him. The new side of the mountain was not sun-parched and hot like the other side. It had shade trees, grassy knolls swaying in a pleasant breeze, various fragrant wild flowers, and even a bench half way up to sit on and enjoy the view of the beautiful green valley on this side of the mountain.

Not long after the old pathway was abandoned, it could no longer be distinguished from the natural tundra and parched landscape on that side of the mountain. Since the weight and energy of the monk no longer affected the ground over the pathway, the local plants and shrubs began to grow up and over it, and soon the pathway disappeared. Inside the monk's mind, only a very faint memory of the old pathway remained.

This is very much the same way thought and thought patterns are held onto and/or let go of in the human mind. When you rehearse a thought it perpetuates itself, and when you completely withdraw a repetitive thought it fades away. When this first happens, the mind seems to yearn for the familiarity and ease of the old, worn path. But, like acquiring any new skill, all it takes is practice, practice, and more practice. Soon your mind will be preoccupied with the new path and the old path will be forgotten.

Like the monk who forged a new path up the other side of the mountain, you will have to put a lot of effort into changing your thought patterns. You have to force yourself to dwell on the positive thoughts and not allow destructive thoughts to distract you. Becoming the master of your conscious mind may not be an easy or quick skill to acquire, but the process really can be simple. Most people do not use their minds as a tool; they allow their minds to use them because they identify with their thoughts and perpetuate the belief that they are their minds. They become prisoners of their thought patterns, feelings, and behaviors. Remember, as I discussed previously, most feelings are direct results of your thoughts and, if you are feeling bad, you can usually trace the feeling back to the initiating thought and change it if appropriate. By honing the ability to change your thought pattern, you can alter negative thoughts by replacing them with positive ones, allowing you to control both your mind and your feelings to a greater extent. This range of control will also extend to the physical body, as we have already seen that the mind and the body are connected.

I am not suggesting you choose to think irrational thoughts, put on rose-colored glasses, or live in a state of blissful denial. There are times when an appropriate thought will result in pain and displeasure. It is part of life. I am suggesting that you be sure you are thinking informed, correct, appropriate, reality-based thoughts as often as you can. I seriously doubt there is anyone who can monitor and control every waking thought, as random or unwanted thoughts will naturally come and go as they pass through the fibers of your mind.

However, you can use your mind like a sieve and choose only to catch and hold onto the constructive thoughts while filtering out the destructive ones. New and healthy thoughts need to be rehearsed and practiced in order to become a part of your cerebral/cognitive biology. Once they do, they manifest in your life like liberating soldiers taking over an oppressed country, setting all new laws and boundaries that are just and fair and allowing freedom and peace to reign in triumph and glory.

Choosing a psychotherapy modality that appeals to you can help you enhance your control over your thoughts and speed up your recovery.

Use psychotherapy for process-efficiency, education, stabilization, and laying the foundation for a prosperous future. Keep in mind a simple formula: name it, claim it, and dump it. Name it by educating yourself with the correct terminology so you can acknowledge, identify, and deal with your experiences and how you feel about them. Claim it by taking responsibility for yourself and your life, by owning and correcting what needs to be healed. Dump it by letting it go and moving forward after you have done this hard work.

If you choose psychotherapy, be goal oriented and "get off the boat when you arrive." When you have been in therapy for a year or two, a good therapist will have made sure you have learned enough to take over managing your own life and will see that you have increased your ability to handle things in a healthy way. Do not become dependent on psychotherapy or use it as a way to avoid taking on the responsibility of applying what you have learned to your life.

Taking control over your life and your illness will plug the energy hemorrhage that has been draining your energy into the black hole of helplessness and hopelessness. Taking control will increase your energy and strength simply because your body will no longer be depleted by things beyond the effects of chronic FMS, which already compromises your energy and strength. Unresolved psychological issues, lack of boundaries, being in a close relationship with a severely dysfunctional person, handing control of your illness over to others, and the ongoing sense of helplessness and hopelessness that all this creates can be far more draining than you may be aware of.

Knowledge is power, and when chronic FMS has taken control over your life by taking away your power to live it as you once did, you can take much of it back by taking charge of what you can – your condition, your life, and your conscious mind. It may not be an easy task in that it will require change, commitment, and practice, but it can be a simple one.

9) Self- Hypnosis — Many people defer from self-hypnosis because they buy into the myth that, when hypnotized, one loses control. In reality, in a state of natural self- hypnosis you do not lose control of your mind. You cannot be hypnotized against your wishes and you can wake yourself up any time. In fact, under hypnosis you are in complete control of your mind. It is so gentle and commonplace, it seems disappointing to people who expect something mystical to happen. The truth is that if you find yourself in a deep daydream, you are in a state of natural hypnosis. In a state of natural hypnosis your breathing and heartbeat slows down and the muscles in the body feel profoundly relaxed. Natural self-

hypnosis is similar to meditation with the exception that in meditation there is no predetermined goal, while the purpose of self-hypnosis is to achieve a specific goal: to contact the subconscious mind directly and deliver positive and non-limiting messages.

Replacing negative messages with positive ones will allow you to experience and enjoy an appropriate level of self-esteem and confidence. Most people behave according to their basic "belief system," whether it is true and rooted in fact or not. This belief system which was formed early in their life by their families, environments and cultures can often produce a distorted and negative self-image. Fortunately, this can be corrected through natural self-hypnosis.

To begin a session of self-hypnosis all you need is twenty uninterrupted minutes and a comfortable chair or bed to relax on. There is no need for candles, bells, whistles, bongs, or chimes. Your intention is to relax mentally and physically, improve self-confidence, improve sleep, and heal your mind and body. There are six easy steps to natural self-hypnosis.

Six easy steps to natural self-hypnosis

- Close your eyes and begin to gently tense and relax small groups of muscles, beginning with the feet and slowly moving up the body, ending with the scalp. During this process you will become aware of where you are holding tension and release it. Because the body and mind are connected, relaxing the body will help free the mind.
- Without raising your head, open your eyes and fix them on a spot on the ceiling slightly above eye level and begin counting backwards from five hundred. Count to yourself silently and do not get stuck if you loose count. Just pick up anywhere you like because you will not be counting for long. This procedure tires your eyes and soon they will close again in their own time. Occupying your conscious mind in this way will allow easier access to your unconscious.
- Give yourself permission to improve the quality of your hypnosis by allowing yourself to fall into a deeper state of mental and physical relaxation. Imagine yourself feeling as heavy and warm as you can.
- Use your natural creative ability to imagine yourself in a beautiful, well tended garden so that you are able to experience an inner state of peace and tranquility in a safe setting.
- Picture yourself feeling confident, fit, and healthy, exactly the way you want to be. Begin directing short, positive messages to your receptive subconscious mind. Your subconscious will accept these affirmations and will act upon them in ways that will affect positive changes within you.

• Count backwards from ten to one and tell yourself that when you reach one you will feel awake, fully alert, rested, and refreshed. This will gently awaken you from your hypnotic state, but if you should fall asleep you will simply awake from an ordinary sleep naturally.

When you are choosing your affirmations, keep them simple and direct them to categories of self-confidence, better sleep, and better health. State clearly the changes you would like to make and guide your subconscious to hear these messages by repeating them a few times. If you are having difficulty getting into a deep state of relaxation you can utilize a number of helpful visualizations, such as: Imagine yourself entering an elevator at the top of a building that is going down. As you descend, watch the indicator as the car passes by each floor and, as the elevator slowly falls to the bottom, feel yourself sinking into a deeper state of hypnosis. Or, imagine yourself watching a pendulum swinging back and forth. Begin slowing down the rhythm of the pendulum while you are telling yourself you are sinking deeper into hypnosis. Or, imagine yourself slowly walking down a staircase seeming to have no end while telling yourself that, with each step you take, you are going into a deeper and more relaxing state of hypnosis.

Experiencing a deep, relaxing state of natural self-hypnosis on a daily basis while practicing positive affirmations will not only help you feel more confident and relaxed in life, it can ease the stresses and tensions that contribute to physical body pain. With practice, you will eventually learn to enter a state where you feel as though you have left your body and are floating a little above it, away from the pain.

In this way you can dissociate yourself from pain for as long as your session lasts, while at the same time delivering positive messages to you unconscious mind. Following this by a relaxing sleep will provide a deeper level of sleep that will be more healing and restorative. When you live with chronic pain, restorative sleep can be very hard to get and anything you can do to promote it is worth your while.

10) Self-Talk Therapy — Aaron Beck, M.D, professor of psychiatry at the University of Pennsylvania, pioneered a simple and effective self-help version of cognitive therapy. His entire focus involves awareness of negative thoughts by writing them down and taking a rational look at how they truthfully match up to reality. This process takes a bit of work, but it can change your distorted beliefs by correcting them so you do not experience their negative consequences. He developed a seven-step technique.

Seven-step technique:

- Put distance between yourself and your negative thoughts by writing all of your thoughts down.
- Identify the things that are bothering you.
- Identify the negative emotions you are feeling.
- Identify the negative thoughts that created the negative emotions.
- Identify distorted perceptions and substitute them with rational responses.
- Reconsider your reactions and determine if, when viewed from a rational point of view, you are justified in being upset.
- Plan corrective action that will solve the problem.

Author David Burns, M.D. has written a number of books about different types of distorted thought patterns leading to negative emotions. He has identified nine common types of distorted thinking.

Nine types of distorted thought patterns:

- All or nothing thinking.
- Labeling with negative terms.
- Overgeneralizations, such as "always" and "never."
- Mental filtering, as in dwelling on the negative.
- Discounting the positive or never being satisfied with the positive things in life.
- Jumping to conclusions.
- Exaggeration.
- Emotional reasoning.
- Self blame.

If you honestly analyze your thought patterns you can identify and untwist your distorted thinking habits. In popular psycho-terminology these distorted thought patterns are commonly referred to as "stinking-thinking" or "catastrophic thinking."

When you are breaking yourself of the stinking-thinking habit, Dr. Burns suggests that you talk to yourself like you would talk to a best friend. Fully examine the evidence and try to see the big picture. Take a look at how your negative thinking about yourself in one area may influence your behavior in another. Look for partial successes in your experiences, or what some call the "silver lining" or the "gift in the garbage." Take a survey of a situation you are experiencing and see if your response is justified. Define the terminology you use to describe a situation and see if it is realistic.

If something is bothering you, find a way to solve the problem. If it cannot be solved, find a way to accept it and move on. It may seem like all of these bits of advice are too simplistic, but even if you exercise a small degree of awareness about your thinking patterns you will improve your responses to situations and avoid a lot of unnecessary negativity. Learning to use the self-talk method of cognitive therapy can help you lift the veil of depression and reduce the pain that accompanies negative thinking.

Eye Movement Desensitization & Reprocessing (EMDR)

Francis Shapiro of the Mental Research Institute Inc. in Palo Alto, California provided a summary of EMDR that is succinct and clear, "The use of saccadic eye movements (rapid left to right movement) for treating post-traumatic stress disorder (PTSD) is described. The procedure involves eliciting from clients sequences of large-magnitude, rhythmic saccadic eye movements while holding in the mind the most salient aspect of a traumatic memory." This process has several results, including:

- Lasting reduction of anxiety.
- Changes in cognitive assessment of a memory.
- Cessation of flashbacks, intrusive thoughts and sleep disturbances.

The summary continues, "The procedure can be extremely successful in only one session as indicated by a previous controlled study and a case history presented. It does not require a hierarchical approach as in desensitization or the elicitation of disturbingly high levels of anxiety over a prolonged period of time, as in flooding."

The use of EMDR as a means of neutralizing PTSD has been very successful in controlled studies and in treatment of patients and is continually being refined. Post-traumatic stress disorder can be a disabling condition characterized by a number of symptoms, such as: anxiety; sleep disturbances; flashbacks; disturbing and intrusive thoughts related to a traumatic event; and a variety of irrational beliefs, such as low self-esteem. Sexual assault and molestation victims and war veterans are two of the largest groups susceptible to this disorder.

In both groups, traumatic memories seem to be central to the manifestation of their symptoms. Other forms of trauma causing PTSD, such as traumatic childhood memories, the accumulated effects of a long-term abusive relationship, or a traumatic accidental injury, can also be treated by this innovative therapy. EMDR involves requiring some form of exposure to traumatic memories to allow desensitization to take place, while maintaining a cognitive reassessment in terms that redefine and assign a new meaning to these events, thereby alleviating self blame.

Desensitization and reprocessing are both relevant aspects of neutralizing the negative effects of PTSD. A single session of EMDR can be sufficient to completely desensitize traumatic memories, dramatically change cognitive self-assessments, and significantly relieve anxiety. Francine Shapiro accidentally discovered the positive effects of saccadic eye movements on PTSD sufferers while she was treating her own intrusive and disturbing thoughts.

Her discovery has evolved into a procedure requiring the client to keep in mind one or more of the following:

- A visual image of the memory.
- The negative assessment of the trauma, including a negative self-statement.
- The physical anxiety response.

While the client focuses on these items the therapist will elicit multiple saccadic eye movements by asking them to follow a repeated side-to-side movement of the therapist's finger. The therapist holds up an index finger about twelve inches in front of the client's face and asks them to follow it as it is moved back and forth. The finger is moved rapidly and rhythmically, from extreme right to extreme left, across the client's line of vision at a rate of two back-and-forth movements per second over a distance of twelve inches. The therapist's finger repeatedly moves back-and-forth twelve to twenty four times in one set of saccades.

During this session, if the client cannot keep in mind all three aspects representing the traumatic event simultaneously in their consciousness, the presence of any one of them can be sufficient to achieve full desensitization. If one set of saccades is not enough to completely desensitize the client from being disturbed by the memory, they are asked to clear their mind completely (blank out the picture), take a deep breath, and repeat the process. The client is then asked if the picture and the feeling attached to it has changed. If the anxiety level does not decrease, the client is asked if the picture has changed or if another memory has popped up, and another set of saccades can be repeated if necessary.

Oftentimes, one session will neutralize an entire tangled glob of traumatic memories in one fell swoop. This is because all of our memories are stored in the same place in the brain. When you fully access and release the negative energy stored from the memory of one traumatic event, the energy from other traumas processes out along with it, much like a drop of rain-water collects other drops as it naturally slides down a window along its way. This energy-releasing process can go on for weeks, and even a few months, after only one session of EMDR has ended.

The energy discharged from the brain into the body from a traumatic event can feel a bit strange and cause mild effects in the body. During the one session I had, I felt a sudden, mild jolt or energy surge throughout my body which lasted for a few seconds. It was not at all painful, but felt quite strange. The next morning when I woke up the skin on my upper eyelids was red and a little sore, like I had been out in the sun a bit too long the previous day. Over the next few days the skin dried up and lightly pealed away, just like it would have from moderate sunburn.

I continued to experience waves of mild feelings that felt like soothing molasses pouring over my body from the top of my head down to my toes. I eventually noticed I was no longer plagued by negative intrusive thoughts during the day, nor was I being kept awake by traumatic flashbacks in bed at night. I was still able to pull up my most traumatic memories, but it took a considerable amount of effort to do so and, when I saw them, I did not relive them anymore. In fact they seemed far away, small, and inconsequential. I was elated. The EMDR worked just as it was explained to me and was very successful in just one session. I believe it continued to work for several months as I processed out a lifetime of traumatic memories from my subconscious mind, mostly in my dreams.

When desensitization is successful, negative and intrusive thoughts disappear almost completely and, when they are deliberately retrieved, they are no longer disturbing. After completing desensitization, cognitive therapy is very useful in reprocessing (redefining) negative and inappropriate terms that are part of the irrational beliefs associated with PTSD. Self blame can be eliminated, an appropriate level of self-esteem can be restored, and new, healthier beliefs rooted in reality can be adopted.

EMDR therapy has been refined to include the use of an "Audioscan Unit," a low voltage machine with wires connecting to hand held probes and a headset. When you are ready to begin a session, the therapist gives you a small probe to hold in each hand and a headset to place over your ears. You then follow the same instructions from the first procedure and, instead of following a finger to induce a set of saccades, the therapist turns on the Audioscan Unit.

You experience a light vibrating pulse in one hand alternating to the other in a rhythmic pattern. Then you simultaneously hear a tone pulse in one ear and then the other, which is synchronized with the pulses felt from the hand held probes. These are experienced in unison while you concentrate on the images, feelings, and messages from a traumatic memory. The session is then evaluated in the same way as the saccades eyes movement method until full desensitization is achieved.

The EMDR Training Institute is located on 54 Penny Lane in Watsonville, CA 95076. Their phone number is (831) 372-3900. If you are interested in trying a session of EMDR and you cannot find a practitioner in your area trained in administering the procedure, you can call them and get a list of qualified therapists in your area. If your therapist is interested in learning more about this therapy they can either call the EMDR Institute for information, or go on line to www.Neurotekcorp.com where the Audioscan Unit is sold.

When I opted for EMDR my therapist used the Audioscan Unit on me and it was enormously effective and successful. Four years later the results are the same. I am still enjoying lasting peace from the traumatic memories from my childhood, adolescence and early adulthood that had plagued my conscious mind throughout my adult life. The terror and trauma of chronic FMS was another source of PTSD I needed to neutralize. Now I can sleep peacefully. I no longer blame myself for this illness and I believe I can handle whatever life deigns to throw my way. I will keep on moving forward, always forward.

Homeopathy (Classical/Constitutional)

The science of classical constitutional homeopathy was founded by an eighteenth century German physician, Samuel Hahnemann (1755– 1843). Homeopathy became extremely popular in the U.S. from the late 1970's on, and today offers a real, solid alternative to regular medicine. Hahnemann studied at Leipzig, Germany, where he practiced medicine for ten years. During this time he observed that a specific medicine administered to a healthy person would produce similar symptoms to those of the illness it was intended to cure.

It was from this observation that Dr. Hahnemann developed his "law of similars," around which he developed his system of homeopathy. He published his homeopathic drug catalog, "Reine Arzneimittellehre" (Precept of Pure Drugs), in 1811. Hahnemann developed all of his homeopathic medicines from nature, deriving roughly 80% of them from plants and the others from animals and minerals. These medicines are now called remedies and, because they are all natural, they are among the safest preparations known to medical science. When administered properly, they do not commonly cause side effects and they do not need a doctor's prescription.

Homeopathic remedies are also safe to use in conjunction with most allopathic chemical preparations because they do not interact or interfere with them. The reason for this is the high dilution factor in the potentialization process used to create the final preparations. This means that the remedies do not contain any of the substances they are made from. For instance, a low 30c dose of a homeopathic remedy contains a ratio of one molecule of the substance it is made from to a zillion trillion molecules of distilled water or alcohol used in the dilution process, requiring a container the size of the earth! However, there are some allopathic drugs that interfere with homeopathic remedies because they are so violent they knock the remedy out of the body, or "antidote the remedy," rendering it inactive. The most common of these are anesthesia, antibiotics, and cortisone.

Because these remedies are natural and are progressively diluted, the body does not detect their presence the way it does chemical pharmaceuticals. A remedy is like a silent, invisible spy that can infiltrate the entire body undetected, maintain strength under the right conditions, and continue to do its work undisturbed. Therefore, one dose has the potential of remaining effective for up to two years. Conversely, synthetic drugs bombard the body with foreign, unnatural substances that are quickly detected. The body responds by trying to eliminate them as quickly as possible, creating various side effects and requiring re-dosing every few hours.

Drugs taken in this way can become extremely costly, while homeopathic remedies are very inexpensive. Furthermore, while homeopathy seeks to stimulate the body's ability to heal itself in specific ways, conventional drugs can be harmful because they seek to suppress symptoms that are known to be the body's natural defenses at work. In doing so, they can rob the body of the opportunity to develop its own natural immunity while hampering the body's ability to heal itself. In addition to this, administering a drug that suppresses the body's natural healing mechanisms creates side effects that from a pharmacological perspective are not really side effects at all, but the direct manifestations of synthetic drug symptom suppression.

The term homeopathy represents the law of similars and is derived from the Greek words "*homoios*," meaning similar, and "*pathos*," meaning disease or suffering. The remedies are carefully matched to the patient's overall presentation of symptoms. Today, the homeopathic law of similars is occasionally used in conventional medical therapies, such as immunizations and allergy treatments.

Homeopathy works with the body's natural defenses, rather than against them. Both homeopaths and modern physiologists alike recognize that disease symptoms represent the body's best effort to defend itself and adapt to infections, stress, or injury. Because the body is sometimes unsuccessful in averting the negative effects of every disturbance, it is important to find a natural substance that can mimic the symptoms the person is experiencing to aid the body in defending and curing itself.

Homeopathy has two underlying principles:
- The natural state of the human body is one of health.
- The body possesses the natural ability to heal itself.

Homeopathy is administered on three levels of therapy:
- First aid therapy – for common household injuries.
- Acute therapy – for acute health problems, such as colds, the flu, and injuries.
- Constitutional therapy – for chronic, long-term health problems.

Classical Homeopathy is composed of two highly systematic methods:
- Toxicology-- when the homeopath discovers the specific physical, emotional, and mental symptoms that various substances cause in large doses.
- Case taking-- when the homeopath interviews the patient in great detail to discover the combined physical, emotional, and mental symptoms experienced.

The homeopath then seeks to match the symptoms a patient has to the substance that would cause those same symptoms in a healthy person. Given in small doses, this substance is used to elicit a healing response, to subtly strengthen the body and bring it back into balance. This challenging system of treatment is reliant upon a complete and profound understanding of the awesome complexity of the human being. It holds to the philosophy that the mind and body are not separate, but are one organism, making homeopathy a "holistic" approach that considers the state of the whole individual– physical, mental, and emotional– whereas conventional medicine is often only concerned with the physical manifestations of illness.

Three aspects of the latest homeopathic model for health and disease:
- The wound – an inherited sensitivity or an early life trauma.
- The wall – the adaptive changes that are created to protect or compensate for the wound and are made up of physical symptoms and mental/emotional tendencies.
- The mask – the persona or public self that is presented to the outside world.

The theory behind this model is that it takes enormous energy to produce and maintain the wall and the mask, and this can drain the body of the energy and vitality needed to resist or fight off ailments and disturbances. The administration of the correct homeopathic remedy stimulates the production of vital core energy. This subsequently begins to reorganize the system, heal the wound, and dissolve the wall and the mask. The goal of homeopathic treatment is to return the body to a state of homeostasis with a sense of renewed health, an increase in energy, and a new-found freedom from adaptations and limitations.

The first two levels of homeopathic therapy are for treating first aid and acute conditions that can respond to the correct remedy quickly, effectively, and safely; however, these remedies can interfere with the third level therapy that uses a constitutional remedy. Always check with your homeopath before administering a homeopathic remedy at home, especially if you are being treated for a chronic condition with a constitutional remedy. This form of treatment must be administered by a licensed classical homeopath. During this treatment, visits to the homeopath will be more frequent for the first six months (once every two or three months) up to two years and then taper off in frequency as the patient becomes healthier (once every four or five months).

No matter how complex the case, when a remedy is working the patient may not need to be evaluated sooner than every two to three months. Bear in mind that a constitutional remedy acts more slowly than first aid or acute remedies because it is healing a long-term condition on a very deep level through many layers. How long a constitutional remedy will actually take to heal a chronically diseased organism depends on the unique individual, the duration and depth of the disease, and the strength of the immune system at the time treatment begins. I would also like to add that it also depends on the state of alignment of the spinal column.

When treating chronic illness homeopathically, a course of constitutional treatment can range from a few treatments over a few months or years to a lifetime. When a patient with a chronic ailment is initially given the correct constitutional remedy, they may experience what is called a "healing crisis," or a temporary worsening of symptoms. A healing crisis may last for up to two to three weeks.

This is the desired indicator that the remedy is working to stimulate the body's healing process and should be carefully monitored by your homeopath. When the healing crisis is over and your system has re-balanced itself, the healing process becomes subtler, is more gradual, and ongoing. If the substance is not a match, the remedy will not work in this way and another remedy will be tried.

Because side effects are so uncommon in homeopathy, if the wrong remedy is given, either nothing happens at all or the presentation of symptoms becomes clearer, which in turn makes the correct remedy more obvious. It usually does not take too many tries to get the right substance and an experienced homeopath can often pick the correct remedy the first time. Ongoing homeopathic care can also be an effective preventative measure against an unforeseen ailment, and it can ensure deep healing continues to take place in your immune system, increase your overall general health, and help maintain your mental and emotional health.

In order for homeopathy to work you must be committed and patient. You will need to follow specific rules to enable the remedy to continue acting. There are several ways to deactivate, or "antidote," a remedy. Antidoting your remedy can derange or derail your case and bring about a relapse, which can be a quiet return of only a few old symptoms or a loud return of all your symptoms. Getting the case back on track after an antidote can be tricky, as it can take several months and can make the healing process lengthy. To prevent antidoting your remedy, there are a number of substances and treatments you must avoid.

To keep your remedy working, your homeopath will give you a complete list of the substances and treatments to avoid before you are given a remedy. The most common things to avoid are: coffee in any form; certain herbal teas; decaffeinated products; Chinese herbs; all camphor and menthol products; recreational drugs; dental work; electric blankets; mineral hot springs; ultrasound and radiation; air travel in the first month of treatment; strong fumes of any kind; aromatic substances, such as pine, eucalyptus, and rosemary; combination homeopathic remedies; acupuncture; and high levels of stress. All of these will lower the resonance of the homeopathic remedy and interfere with or completely neutralize its effectiveness.

The sophisticated system of evaluating a patient used by Homeopathic Remedy is referred to as the "Laws and Principles of Cure." To my knowledge, conventional medicine does not use any principle involving the word "cure." Its primary concern regarding chronic illness is symptom management and suppression through the use of strong synthetic drugs. The primary concern of homeopathic medicine is to exact a cure through the use of a remedy made from a substance found in nature that is matched as precisely as possible to the patient as a whole and works on an ongoing basis to stimulate the body to heal itself in specific ways.

These remedies that come from plants, animals, and minerals are prepared by grinding the active ingredient (the substance) and mixing it with alcohol and distilled water, then allowing it to soften and steep. This liquid is filtered to produce the base, or "mother tincture," and is then "potentized" through a delicate process of progressive diluting and shaking, which decreases the concentration while increasing the healing power of the medicine. This process continues until the desired potency is attained. Other diluting agents, such as glycerin and lactose, can also be used.

Homeopathic remedies come in various potencies and are manufactured through the specific pharmacological procedure of "potentization," beginning with the base tincture that has the given strength of 1x. To manufacture 2x potency, one part of the base tincture is mixed with nine parts of a mixing agent, such as alcohol or water, and then shaken vigorously ten times. To manufacture 3x potency, one part of the 2x potency is mixed with nine parts of the diluting agent and vigorously shaken ten times again, and so on until the desired potency is attained.

In addition to "x" potencies, there are also "c" potencies that are prepared the same way, except they are mixed at a ratio of ninety-nine to one, instead of nine to one. There is also "k" potency with a ratio of one thousand to one. A potency of 1,000k is labeled 1m and 10,000k potency is labeled 10m, and so on. The process of potentization can continue anywhere from vigorously shaking a single time to over one million times. Homeopathic medicines (remedies) are most commonly potentized to measurements of three, six, twelve, thirty, one hundred, and two hundred. These remedies are labeled: 6x, 12x, 30x, 6c, 12c, 30c, l00c, 200c, and so on.

The science of homeopathy has become so refined, homeopaths have discovered that the more a homeopathic medicine has been potentized the longer it will act, the deeper it will act, and the fewer doses will generally be needed. Although this is so, it has not entirely been explained. However, a 1990's British Medical Journal reported that, "the amount of positive evidence in the best studies showing the success of this method of treatment have been sufficient to establish homeopathy as an indicated treatment for certain conditions."

The remedies are commonly administered in small round sugar pills that have been coated with the medicinal substance and are placed underneath the tongue until they are dissolved. Remedies can also be administered in powder or liquid form as well, and are created in licensed homeopathic laboratories under the strictest of quality controls.

The resonance of a homeopathic remedy is an energetic vibration that is much like the energy your body produces naturally. It is the "good vibration" that stimulates your body to heal itself by mimicking what is called a "distortion signal," which is produced by an energetic imbalance from the hypothalamus. The hypothalamus is the grand central station of the brain because it controls so many major biological functions and systems.

This distortion signal is manifested in the body and the mind in the form of symptoms and disease. When a distortion signal is met and mimicked by the energy of a remedy given in a minute, potentized dose, the distortion signal will begin to shrink while the body is simultaneously stimulated to naturally heal itself. This process supports the body's natural ability to heal itself physically, mentally, and emotionally, and energetically brings the whole person back into balance. This process begins on a cellular level as the body literally rebuilds itself from the ground up.

The cells of the body are directed by our DNA to replace themselves in cycles. This means our bodies are constantly rebuilding themselves according to DNA directives, which can be positively or negatively influenced by our current state of overall health. For instance, when we suffer certain traumas or stressors, a genetic weakness in our DNA can be triggered and manifest itself as an illness. Furthermore, our DNA strands must be rebuilt and replaced from time to time and are constantly being monitored and patrolled by proteins and amino acids, which act as emergency repair crews.

Underneath the DNA strand is the energy pattern of the living body, or the "life-force energy," found in all living things. It is this energy pattern that the DNA strand is reliant upon to rebuild itself. The resonance of homeopathic medicines work to fortify the very energy pattern our DNA strand uses to replace itself. The theory is that, if given enough time, homeopathic remedies can strengthen our DNA and even heal inherent genetic weaknesses.

Nutrition

Research has shown that our food is lacking in sufficient nutrition to maintain the proper balance of nutrients for necessary energy production. Today in the U.S., our soils are depleted of minerals and are said to contain only 20% of the nutrients that they did in the 1940's. The combination of this inferred nutritional bankruptcy, stress, and the presence of toxins in our environment have been linked to a host of illnesses, such as cancer, FMS, lupus, arthritis, allergies, and a weakened immune system.

Therefore, introducing a nutritional protocol into daily life is necessary to fortify the body by enhancing its natural healing ability and improving energy production. This can be done in two ways: by the use of nutritional supplements and through our diet. Although this may not be a curative measure for many chronic conditions, including a nutritional protocol in your healing combination can raise your level of functioning and overall health.

Adding exercise to your daily routine will enhance the benefits of any nutritional protocol and is absolutely necessary when battling conditions such as chronic illness and obesity. The epidemic of obesity in the U.S. is caused by: eating too much of the wrong foods for the wrong reasons; eating foods that are nutritionally bankrupt and cause you to crave even more of these foods; not enough exercise; too much stress; genetic predisposition; and a build up of systemic and environmental toxins. Overeating causes a build up of metabolic toxins that clog the liver, hampering its ability to filter the toxins and create the enzymes (prostaglandins) essential in controlling the production of serotonin and dopamine, which are responsible for creating energy and a sense of well-being.

The result of low levels of serotonin and dopamine is a dramatic drop in energy production, an increase in depression and fatigue, and food cravings. Proper nutrition enables the body to produce the energy necessary to heal itself from the ravages of the day through restorative sleep. However, because of the pain, fatigue, and depression inherent in chronic FMS, the body cannot produce enough energy in one night's sleep to heal itself from the daily affects of this illness. Furthermore, FMS symptoms cause numerous sleep disturbances, which prevent restorative sleep from occurring.

Any fortification you can provide the body in the form of nutrition, especially nutrition that specifically helps your body produce more energy, will help alleviate the pain, fatigue, and depression that prevents restorative sleep. When energy deficit is a major problem, as it is with chronic FMS, the body simply cannot get ahead of the destructive effects of this disease. Try as it may, the body can barely hold on to its basic living functions, and can do little more than tread water.

While management therapies can only pull you out of the water into a slowly sinking boat, alleviating your symptoms temporarily. They cannot fix the proverbial hole in the bottom of your boat. Metaphorically, they can only help you bail out the water; they can do nothing to plug up and repair the hole causing the leak. Continuous bailing may help to keep you afloat, but it will quickly exhaust you and deplete your energy.

Adding a nutritional protocol to your life by modifying your diet and taking the right supplements is absolutely necessary if you want to aid your body in its efforts to heal FMS. There are countless diets and nutritional protocols available, so in the next section I will go over the ones that will benefit patients who suffer from chronic FMS.

Specific Nutritional Protocols

Meyers Cocktail

"The Meyers Cocktail" is named after its creator, the late John Meyers, MD, of Baltimore, Maryland. This nutritional boost comes from an intravenous micronutrient treatment containing magnesium, calcium, vitamin B complex, and vitamin C. It has been used in the treatment of chronic FMS for over 25 years and, according to a study published in Alternative Medicine Review 2002; 7(5): 389-403, is safe and effective in promoting and improving the production of cellular energy (ATP). Nutritionist Virginia Hadley, RN from the Tahoma Clinic in Kent, Washington, said, "We have had good clinical success with this treatment to reduce pain and promote detoxification."

In 2006, Yale University researchers tested the Meyers Cocktail on forty chronic FMS patients in a controlled double-blind study. Once a week, for eight weeks, they injected participants with 37mls of nutrients through a large syringe (about 7 teaspoons). The injections were given very slowly over a period of twenty minutes. The study measured tender points, depression levels, and quality of life. David Katz, MD, associate clinical professor of epidemiology and public health at Yale University, reported, "This three-month pilot study showed significant improvement in all pertinent outcome measurements with the Meyers Cocktail and none with the placebo solution. Our results strongly suggest that Meyers Cocktail may well offer therapeutic benefit in chronic fibromyalgia."

D-Ribose

Rest and sleep alone cannot compensate for the energy deficit of chronic FMS. No matter how much someone with chronic FMS rests, they never seem to have enough energy. The chronic fatigue of fibromyalgia is caused by the body's inability to make enough ATP (energy molecules). D-ribose is the key building block used in the cell matrixes that produce naturally occurring ATP. The ATP energy molecules in the body are made up of ribose, B vitamins, and phosphate.

Our body acquires ribose through its metabolism of glucose in food; however, this process is very slow and cannot always keep up with restoring the energy that is lost. It can take several days to restore the lost ATP of one day in the life of a healthy person, and much longer for someone with chronic FMS. Studies done in 2006 have shown that supplementing the diet with D-Ribose can dramatically increase the rate in which the body replenishes ATP in patients with chronic fibromyalgia.

Scientists now know supplementing with ribose can reduce muscle pain, stiffness, and exercise fatigue and that people tolerate it well with no side effects. Jacob Teitelbaum, MD and Medical Director of Maryland's Annapolis Center for Effective Chronic Fatigue Syndrome/ Fibromyalgia Therapies, conducted a ribose study in 2006. Chronic FMS patients were given five grams (5,000mg) of ribose three times a day for twenty-eight days. The results reported that, "In just twelve days, sixty-six percent of those taking ribose had significant improvement in energy, sleep, mental clarity, and pain intensity with a forty-four percent average increase in energy, and an overall thirty percent increase in well-being."

You can find D-Ribose in powdered form, usually in containers of either 100gms or 200gms. It is easy to mix with juice and the recommended dosage is only one half of a teaspoon prior to exertion, such as exercise or an outing. You can safely use it as needed to improve your level of energy and functioning. Athletes that need extra energy prior to exerting themselves or need to recover quickly afterwards commonly use ribose. I have used it and found it very effective.

Special Dietary Supplemental

In addition to specific nutritional supplements aimed at improving production of energy in the body, there are many other supplemental products on the market that have been met with great success. These products can be purchased over the Internet, in some chiropractic offices, and through sales representatives. To name a couple, a company called IS-AGENIX sells nutritional supplements for men and women, and two body cleansing programs that include nutritional foods. Their website is www.support@isagenix.net. Another very successful company is called 4Life Transfer Factor at www.4life.com on line or you can call them directly at (866) 315-4002 to learn more.

My osteopath takes Transfer Factor and highly recommends it. This nutritional supplement is based on what are called transfer factors, tiny molecules that transfer immunity information from one entity to another, such as between mother and baby during breast-feeding.

Transfer factors educate the immune system to recognize and fight infection, and also help it remember healthy immune functioning. Because transfer factors are not species specific, 4Life has combined transfer factors from bovine (cow) colostrums and egg yolks, which are more effective when combined than when used alone. Because chronic stress can seriously compromise the immune system and drastically affect the production of T-cells (cancer fighting cells), a supplement that supports healthy immune function can be very beneficial for counteracting the negative effects from chronic FMS stress.

There are two types of immunity protecting the human body: The first, innate immunity, is present at birth and provides the first line of defense against microorganisms. The second, adaptive immunity, retains the memory of all the invaders it has faced over time in its battles against infection and disease. Supporting the immune system with a nutritional supplement, such as transfer factors, increases the production and activity of NK cells (natural killer cells) in our adaptive immunity that seek out and destroy invading harmful cells. Results of an independent study conducted at the Russian Academy of Medical Science conclusively showed that, "Transfer Factor Plus Advanced Formula proved to propel NK cell activity to a remarkable 437 percent above normal immune responses." Because not every baby is breast-fed, and because our immune systems are weakened by stress and poor nutrition, borrowing the immune memory from cows and chickens can help our immune systems learn to recognize and respond more effectively to invasion.

There is also a recommended nutritional protocol for chronic fibromyalgia in a publication called "Prescription for Nutritional Healing," written by Phyllis A. Balch, CNC and James F. Balch, MD. Note: This publication does not acknowledge the fact that chronic fatigue syndrome is a symptom of chronic FMS. These protocols are extensive, clearly presented, and include suggestions on vitamin, mineral, and herbal supplements. I have extracted and combined a nutritional supplementation protocol from their suggestions that seems do-able and affordable and has proven to be very effective.

My Nutritional Protocol

- Vitamin A; 24,000 IU daily, for one month, then slowly reduce to10,000 IU daily; a free radical scavenger that protects body cells and enhances the immune system.
- Vitamin B complex; 100 mg 2 X daily; essential for increased energy, normal brain function, healing the central nervous system, and reducing nerve pain. *Do not take B vitamins at bedtime because they are "metabolic cofactor vitamins" and stimulate neurotransmitters in the brain that spark vivid, weird dreams. The best time is at breakfast and dinner with the rest of the twice daily supplements.
- Vitamin C; 1000 mg 2 X daily; antiviral, antioxidant, anti-stress, strengthens the immune system, and helps with energy production.
- Vitamin D; 1200 IU daily; needed for reversing osteoporosis in older women, improving absorption of minerals calcium and phosphorus.
- Vitamin E; 800 IU daily for 1 month, then slowly reduce to 400 IU daily; free radical scavenger (antioxidant), enhances the immune sys-

tem, and reduces hot flashes.

- Calcium citrate with Vitamin D; 1500 mg daily (500mg 3 X day); needed for proper function of muscles, and bone density. Do not take all at once.
- Coenzyme Q;10 75 mg daily; improves oxygen to cells and boosts the immune system.
- Lecithin; 1200 mg 3 X daily; vitamin E and fat emulsifier, promotes energy, enhances the immune system and brain function, improves circulation, acts as an antioxidant, and helps lower cholesterol.
- Magnesium malate; 1000 mg twice daily; relieves muscle spasms and pain and is needed for energy production.
- Multiple vitamins with added minerals; 1 daily.
- Niacin; 500 mg 2 to 3 X daily; use "no-flush niacin" for increased circulation.
- DLPA; 500 mg daily, every other week; relieves pain, elevates mood swings, and increases mental alertness.
- Soy protein; 30 mg daily; natural form of estrogen, relieves hot flashes, protects against heart disease and osteoporosis.
- Flaxseed oil; 14 grams of omega 3,6, and 9 EFAs 1 tbsp. daily; omega-3 promotes production of anti-inflammatory prostaglandins, protects the   body against heart disease and cancer, and prevents constriction of blood and bronchial vessels. It is also an old American Indian remedy for asthma and allergies. Note: An alternative to flaxseed oil is fish oil!
- Fish oil; 2400 mg twice daily; great source of the omegas and recent studies suggest the absorption rate of omega-3 EFAs is higher than that of flaxseed oil!
- Malic acid; at least 800 mg twice day; increases oxygen to muscles, promotes energy, and comes in the form of magnesium malate.
- D-Ribose; 5 gm three times a day at first, and then decrease as desired; Increases energy production in the body, especially when exercise is part of a daily routine.

Note: I do not use MSM because it tends to aggravate my central nervous system and increases nerve pain.

I am still using this protocol today and found that, soon after I began the regime, I felt better and stronger overall. Nutritional supplements have helped my healing process tremendously. They gave me the strength I needed to take on the challenge of reconditioning my body through a series of exercise protocols. If you do some research and poke around your local health food store, you too can find the nutritional supplement protocol that you can afford.

The large chain drug stores often have the lowest prices on nutritional supplements, offer special purchases (ex: buy one/get one free), and discounts with coupons and in-store rebates. In addition to supplements, pay close attention to your diet. Eating the proper foods while taking supplements will maximize your results.

For breakfast, I like to eat a bowl of mixed berries, plain yogurt, a half cup of quinoa cooked cereal or about three tablespoons of flax cereal, half a sliced banana, and about two tablespoons of roasted flax seeds on top. I take my morning vitamins with a drink made of eight ounces water, eight ounces prune or tomato juice, and a heaping tablespoon each of lecithin granules and ground flax. For lunch, I like to have a salad of dark greens, tofu, raw broccoli tops and sprouts, sprinkled with roasted flax seeds and topped with two tablespoons of dressing (usually low-sodium soy sauce with a little flax-seed oil or Italian dressing). To break up the monotony, I often use a can of albacore tuna instead of tofu in my lunch salad. For dinner, I have lean protein with steamed dark veggies or a glass of V8 juice. I snack on fruit and usually drink water or tea (peppermint or sometimes black).

Nutrition for Energy, Healing, and Overall Health

Before I discuss what you should be consuming, I would like to discuss what you should not be consuming and why. Science-based nutrition addresses both issues fully and works with the philosophy that just because you get sick does not mean you are unhealthy. Sickness often strengthens the body's defenses and is necessary in the development of a strong immune system that functions properly. Also, health is not the absence of sickness, but rather the ability to effectively fight off hostile organisms and heal and repair wounds and injuries.

Chronic illness only results when the normal mechanisms of healing and repairing the body have become thwarted for some reason. These reasons can vary, from living with severe stress, such as a job that demands too much or a marriage that is no longer working, to a toxic environment, such as an invasive organism that takes hold, a triggered genetic weakness, or an injury. All these kinds of things can tax the immune system and central nervous system enough to cause an imbalance in the body, which causes our cells to become chronically ill.

The Cells and the Cell Code

There are many different types of cells that make up the body, each of which have special functions. To name a few, muscle cells contract and relax to regulate involuntary breathing, heartbeat, digestion, and the voluntary movement of bones. Glandular cells produce and secrete vital substances, such as mucous, hormones, and hydrochloric acid. The cells of the soft connective tissues and muscles support the movements of the spinal and skeletal matrix. The most complex of the cells are the white blood cells, which circulate freely throughout the body with both random and direct movements.

While some white blood cells engage in hand-to-hand combat with germs and other foreign substances, others produce antibodies (proteins that bind to foreign substances to help destroy them). Many of us remember the evil doctor who took over the micro-sized submarine in the movie "The Fantastic Voyage." In the end, the doctor was killed by giant white corpuscles, which represented white blood cells. White blood cells help protect the body against infection in its immune response and play a role in inflammation and allergic reactions.

There are literally thousands of functions performed by the different cell types in the body. Within this amazing diversity lies the simplicity of what is called the bio-chemical cell code. There appears to be two key components of the cell code: 1) the level of calcium present in the body and 2) the relative levels of chemicals called cyclic nucleotides. The interaction between these two components is what determines the rhythm of the cell.

Although each cell group has a different type of response when called to action, the two elements of their bio-chemical cell code remain the same; only the ratios of these elements vary. The apparent ratio of calcium and cyclic nucleotides places each cell between two extremes of cellular activity: slow or relaxed; fast or hyperactive. Depending on this ratio, the chemical message that puts one cell into fast action may put another cell in slow motion.

All hormones, nerve impulses, most pharmaceuticals, and many poisons work strictly through the cell code. The primary modulator of the cell code comes from three groups of prostaglandins, which are a bio-chemical. Prostaglandins are unsaturated fatty acids that are dissolvable in liquid that resemble hormones in their activity by the way they control smooth muscle contraction, blood pressure, inflammation, and body temperature.

Prostaglandins are responsible for setting the rhythm of the cells by changing the levels of calcium and cyclic nucleotides. Prostaglandins are also responsible for determining how the cells will respond to outside stimulation, thus regulating the body's responses to stress and injury. For instance, when you receive a penetrating wound from the outside, different cells in the body go to work in a harmonic unison. The platelets quickly clump while blood vessels quickly constrict to stop the bleeding.

When infection sets in, blood vessels dilate to increase blood flow to the wound. White blood cells quickly rally and move in to fight the invading organisms, while others slowly multiply and mature into cells that can produce antibodies, then quickly pour out their antibodies to help fight the invaders. When infection is subdued, antibody production slows and white blood cells quickly return to their random travels through the bloodstream, remembering their experience and what they have learned.

Blood vessels remain dilated to deliver oxygen and nutrients to the wound site and let the healing begin. Connective tissue cells quickly lay down fibers to form scar tissue and then slow their activity to prevent keloid formation (too large a scar). The scar then contracts and all that remains in the cells are the memories of the event. The brain remembers the event, the white blood cells remember the germs, and these memories condition the immune response for future assaults of the same kind.

Prostaglandins

As I mentioned before, prostaglandins are the primary modulator of the cell code and control the fast (pro-inflammatory) and slow (anti-inflammatory) rhythms of the body's cellular responses. Prostaglandins represent a key link between what we eat and how our bodies function because they are produced from the unsaturated essential fatty acids (EFAs) in our food. Because prostaglandins play such a vital role in modulating our cellular rhythms, if their production is distorted by a deficiency of EFAs the rhythm of our cellular responses will be off beat, causing our entire body to suffer.

The Center for Genetics, Nutrition and Health, Washington DC, U.S.A reported in 2007 that the human diet has changed drastically over the last 150 years; however, the genetic profile has not significantly changed over the past 10,000 to 15,000 years. Pre-historic humans used to eat foods high in omega-3 EFAs and evolved on a dietary ratio of omega-6 to omega-3 of 1:1. Humans now consume these EFAs at a ratio of omega-6 to omega-3 of 10-20:1 and above. The over-consumption in our western culture of saturated fatty acids from vegetable oils, processed foods, and meat causes a nutritional imbalance that promotes chronic pain and inflammation in the body.

Eating too many saturated fatty acids creates an excess of pro-inflammatory prostaglandins which are the fast cell code modulators, causing nerves to become sensitized to pain. In fact, the very enzymes that convert saturated fatty acids into pro-inflammatory molecules are the targets of drugs used to treat pain and inflammation and carry a significant risk when used on a long-term basis. Therefore, balancing pro-inflammatory and anti-inflammatory prostaglandins through diet becomes essential.

Symphony of Cells

Because of my training in classical music and voice, it is easy for me to visualize the body and its cell action as a symphony of cells. This visualization was sparked by the ideas of Howard Press, MD and Naturopath in Carmel Valley, California. To illustrate my point, image that you are going out for the evening to hear a symphony orchestra play an exquisite suite. The magnificent stage represents the body and the musicians represent the cells grouped by like instruments, each having their own specific sound. The musical score represents the cell code from which they all play. The conductor represents the prostaglandins (essential fatty acids) that regulate the rhythm and speed (the tempo) by which the musicians (the cells) play, be it staccato or largo (fast or slow).

When the curtain rises and the performance begins, the conductor stands tall and balanced, raises his baton, and begins gracefully modulating the tempo of each passage as the score is played. As each group of musicians carefully follows the score, they keep a constant and watchful eye on the conductor for their entrances and tempos as sounds of their instruments come and go throughout the suite. As the conductor cues their entrances and modulates their tempos, the suite is performed in perfect harmony.

However, if the conductor had too many martinis and too little food with his dinner prior to the performance, he will be struggling to stand up, his rhythms will surely be off, and he may even lose his place in the score. The musicians will become disoriented and confused, and some may even stop playing. Thus, the final movement may never be played, the curtain may come crashing down prematurely, and the entire evening will have been a disaster. Chronic illness feels similar to the cacophony produced by such an orchestra, and can happen when the body's prostaglandins are not functioning properly.

Essential Fatty Acids and Prostaglandins

The right ratio between pro-inflammatory and anti-inflammatory prostaglandins comes from consuming high amounts of unsaturated essential fatty acids (EFAs) in the diet. Primordial man ate a diet low in saturated fats and half of the fat he did consume was high in unsaturated fats (essential fatty acids), as the majority of it came from plants, one of its ultimate sources. The vast majority of plants produce two types of EFAs:

1) omega-3 fatty acid/lionolenic acid (LNA) and 2) omega-6 fatty acid/ linoleic acid (LA).

All omega-3 fatty acid is converted by eicospentaenoic acid (EPA) into prostaglandin E-1 (PGE-1), which is mostly anti-inflammatory. The "ideal dietary ratio" of omega-6 to omega-3 is 3:1. It is only when omega-6 fatty acid is ingested in large amounts that it becomes a problem. The American Academy of Pain Management (AAPM) reported in their Practical Guide to Clinicians, "Historical estimates place the ratio of omega-6 to omega 3 at nearly 1:1 for prehistoric humans. By the turn of the century (1900) the ratio had increased to about 4:1 and the current American ratio is about 25:1." The EFA consumption in the Western diet is clearly way out of balance. When there is this kind of excess in omega -6 fatty acid, it is converted by arachidonic acid (AA) into prostaglandin E-2 (PGE-2), which is highly pro-inflammatory.

The AAPM also reported, "Many of the chronic inflammatory conditions that accompany EFA imbalance are currently treated with symptom -specific pharmaceutical drugs such as steroids, prednisone, aspirin and other nonsteroidal anti-inflammatory drugs (NSAIDs). The problem with these drug therapies is they prevent the formation of 'good' anti-inflammatory eicosanoids (PGE-1), or they shift the production of one type of eicosanoid to another (PGE-1 to PGE-2)." This means these drugs either prevent production of anti-inflammatory prostaglandins or they increase production of inflammatory prostaglandins. Both of these actions are pro-inflammatory.

As I discussed earlier, PGE-2 is responsible for the chronic pain caused by the "Omega-6 Arachidonic Cascade into PGE-2." Too much PGE-2 is the biological equivalent of pouring gasoline onto a fire. Even though omega-6 fat is essential to our diet, by simply increasing your intake of omega-3 essential fatty acid you can balance the ratio and inhibit the conversion of excess omega-6 fatty acid into pro-inflammatory PGE-two.

Keep in mind when you read your EFA supplemental label to make sure it contains the recommended counter-balance ratio between omega-6 and omega-3, which is as a 1:3 ratio, or one part of omega-6 to at least three parts of omega-3, plus omega-9/gammaoleic acid (GLA). This "counter-balance ratio" will increase the conversion of omega-3 into PGE -1, a powerful anti-inflammatory agent that will prevent the excess production of pro-inflammatory PGE-2, helping reduce any inflammation existing in the body. Omega-9 should also be present.

Our modern U.S. diet is high in non-essential fatty acids (mostly solid animal fats and synthetic fats) and is sorely deficient in EFAs. This deficiency of EFAs in our diet has a profound negative effect on the way our body makes prostaglandins, resulting in distorting the body's expression of the cell code (i.e. the tight conductor).

Research on the importance of EFAs began in the late 1970's, and today there are thousands of scientific studies showing that EFAs play a critical role in human health and the body's natural anti-inflammatory response. In fact, omega-3 and omega-6 essential fatty acids are so important to the way the body functions that they are the only nutrients the United States Government, the American Heart Association, the World Health Organization, and the British Nutritional Foundation have all agreed to routinely recommend in proportional mega-doses for the maintenance of health and the prevention of disease.

EPA and DHA (The Long-Chain EFAs) Fall Into Two Categories

- Omega-3 derived from plants, such as nuts and flaxseeds that contain a shorter chain fatty acid: alpha-linolenic acid (ALA).
- Omega-3 derived from marine life, such as fish that contain the longer chain fatty acids: eicosapentaenoic acid (EPA) and docosahexaenoic acid (DHA) that are so essential to health maintenance.

While it was once believed that human beings could easily convert plant sources of essential fatty acids (ALA) into EPA and DHA, recent research suggests that only about five percent of ALA actually ends up converting into EPA, and may not easily covert into DHA at all. This suggests that the two omega-3 EFAs found naturally in fish oil (EPA and DHA) may be the most efficient form from which to get these vitally important omega-3 EFAs.

This means if you use a plant-derived omega-3 EFA, such as flaxseed oil, you might want to take one teaspoon three times a day to insure you are getting a therapeutic dose of omega-3s in EPA and DHA.

A Norwegian company called Nordic Naturals sells fish oil that is of the highest purity available. It claims to have no fishy taste and has proven itself in Norway to be the highest in concentration, freshness, and purity by exceeding the stringent Norwegian Medical Standard (NMS) and the European Pharmacopoeia Standard (EPS) for maximum allowances of toxic peroxides, dioxins, PCBs, and the heavy metals mercury and lead, by using testing methods established by the World Health Organization (WHO).

It is important to note that fish oil quality standards do not exist in the U.S.. Nordic Naturals distributes their fish oil products in the U.S. and World markets and can likely be found in your local health food stores.

You can also contact them directly by phone in Watsonville, CA on location at (800) 662-2544, or go on line to order at www.nordicnaturals.com, or get more information at www.omega-research.com. I use it and I like the lovely orange flavor best. It also comes in strawberry.

Since our body is not able to produce omega-3 or omega-6 EFAs, we must make sure we ingest enough of the right foods and supplements in sufficient quantities. Not only for general health maintenance, because in the case of fibromyalgia, EFA's must be ingested in therapeutic quantities. The recommended daily dose of omega-3 EFAs for adults using the ISSFAL international standards is 650mg. A therapeutic dose for adults of omega-3 plus omega-9 would be in the neighborhood of at least 2400mg of fish oil two to three times a day, or two to three teaspoons a day of cold pressed, refrigerated flaxseed oil.

In order to derive prostaglandins from EFAs they must be made active by a series of chemical reactions. They also must be combined with the minerals magnesium, iron, selenium, and zinc and the vitamins biotin, B-3, B-6, C, and E. Deficiencies of these nutrients will adversely affect the formation and production of prostaglandins from those we get in our diet, as do high levels of sugar and non-essential saturated fatty acids.

There are fifty or so prostaglandins in the human body divided into three large groups, PGE-1 from omega-3, PGE-2 from omega-6, and PGE-3 from omega 9. PGE-1 and PGE-3 have a very different effect on the body than PGE-2 prostaglandins. PGE-2 makes the rhythm of our cells fast (which is why it is called pro-inflammatory), while PGE-1 and PGE-3 make the cell rhythm slow (which is why they are called anti-inflammatory). These proven conclusions summarize a phenomenon explained by a vast assortment of data derived from laboratory experiments, public health surveys and the nutritional treatment of sick patients.

The 20th Century diet has laid down a pattern of nutritional deficiency that is common in nearly every kind of human disease, whether it be called heart disease, diabetes, cancer, multiple sclerosis, Crohn's disease, lupus, asthma, schizophrenia, dysmenorrheal, depression, or eczema. For example, studies have shown that schizophrenia has been associated with a ratio of omega-6 to omega-3 of 70:1 (when a healthy ratio is roughly 3:1).

This pattern shows that, while there is a deficiency in the production of anti-inflammatory PGE-1 and PGE-3, there is an extreme excess of production of pro-inflammatory PGE-2. This is largely due to the fact that the production of PGE-1 and PGE-3 becomes significantly blocked by the consumption of sugar, saturated fat, and alcohol and from vitamin and mineral deficiencies in our diet.

These blocks in the production of anti-inflammatory prostaglandins E -1 and E-3 can also be inherited through our DNA. Even so, an inherited block is still subject to the same influences that otherwise unblock the production of these healthy prostaglandins. Research done by Dr. David Horrobin of the Efamol Research Institute has demonstrated this block in the conversion of LA (omega-3/linoleic acid) and GLA (omega-9/gammaoleic acid) into PGE-1 and PGE-3 in patients with allergies and asthma.

In addition, the chronic production and circulation throughout the body of adrenaline and cortisol (two deadly stress hormones), perhaps resulting from living life in the fast lane in our stressful society and certainly from chronic FMS, also block the production of these two essential prostaglandin groups. Conversely, PGE-2 is being produced in excess, due to the high consumption of trans-fatty acids (TFA's) from animal fats and other products that are so common in the average American diet.

Our food choices, the method of food preparation, and vitamin and mineral deficiencies are largely responsible for the nutritional deficits that cause the imbalance in the production of anti-inflammatory prostaglandins E-1 and E-3; however, this can be easily corrected. Vitamin B and magnesium are necessary to properly convert EFAs into prostaglandins, so make sure you are supplementing your diet with these, along with zinc and selenium. Also, include the antioxidant vitamins C and E that act to protect the EFAs in your body from oxidation damage by free radicals.

Lower your intake of saturated fats (fats that are solid at room temperature), such as those found in whole milk and cream, cheese, coconut oil, palm oil, vegetable shortening, and fatty meat. Increase your dietary intake of liquid polyunsaturated fats, primarily omega-3 essential fatty acid. Omega-3 EFA is found in high quantities in cold-water fish, such as salmon, mackerel, halibut, tuna, herring, cod, and sardines and also in flaxseed, hempseed, cattail seed, and walnut oils.

These appear to protect against cardiovascular disease and cancer. Omega 6 EFA is found in high quantities in corn, sunflower, cottonseed, and safflower oils. Finally, avoid trans-fatty acids (TFAs), substances that are artificially created and are not found in nature, such as hydrogenated vegetable oils found in margarine and packaged foods containing trans-fatty acids to increase shelf-life. A good rule of thumb is "do not eat anything that may contain any kind of hydrogenated substance." These also appear to be associated with increased risk of heart disease and cancer. A Harvard Nurse's Study showed that people who consumed large amounts of margarine had a 66% greater risk of heart disease than those who consumed low amounts of margarine or none at all.

EFAs have been demonstrated in studies to lower total cholesterol when it is consumed in high doses because they increase HDL (the good cholesterol that keeps the bad cholesterol LDL in check). The most efficient way to supplement with EFAs is by taking cold-pressed fish oil with longer-chain fatty acids that contain high levels of omega-3. Because fish oil has been shown to have a higher rate of absorption than other forms of omega-3, you do not have to take it in as high a milligram dose as ground flax or flaxseed oil.

I have found the most cost effective way to supplement my diet with the right EFAs in the desired "counter-balancing" ratio is by taking one tablespoon of cold pressed flaxseed oil twice daily as a therapeutic dose, which most likely is sufficient to compensate for its slower absorption rate in comparison to fish oil. One tablespoon of flaxseed oil contains a total of 14 grams (14000 mg) of EFA/polyunsaturated fats; approximately eight grams (8000+ mg) of anti-inflammatory omega-3 (alpha-lenoleic acid), two grams (2000+ mg) of inflammatory omega-6 (lenolenic acid), and three grams (3000+ mg) of anti-inflammatory omega-9 (gammaoleic acid found in almost all animal and vegetable fats). All three of these EFAs are important in the right amounts.

Organic, unrefined, and filtered cold-pressed flaxseed oil comes in a refrigerated 12ounce and 16 ounce bottle, and can be found in most health food stores. Remember that, although the desired dietary ratio of omega-6 to omega-3 plus omega-9 is ideally 3:1, the nutritional counter-balance ratio between omega-6 and omega-3 plus omega-9 is approximately 1:3, or three times the total omega-3 + 9 to counter-balance the high amounts of omega-6 we consume in our western diet.

Whether you choose to supplement your diet with flaxseed oil or fish oil to protect the EFAs from the stress of oxidation in the body, remember that it is mandatory to supplement the diet with vitamin B-3 and B-6 to counteract the anti-B-6 factor in flax, zinc, magnesium, and selenium. Also remember to substantially reduce your intake of sugar, fat, and alcohol, which block the production of anti-inflammatory prostaglandins E-1 and E-3.

Guaranteeing your body the correct nutrients and EFAs in the correct amount and ratio that promotes production of anti-inflammatory prostaglandins will dramatically help in the suppression of allergies, the hormonal regulation of the central nervous system, and the decrease nerve sensitivity to pain by helping break the pain cycle.

The recommended daily amount of ground flaxseed is three to six tablespoons per day, the recommended daily amount of flaxseed oil is one to three tablespoons per day, and the recommended daily amount of fish oil containing at least 1200mg of omega-3 is one gel cap three times a day. You can safely double these recommendations for a therapeutic dose.

Also, snacking on a few sardines or approximately one ounce of mixed nuts daily, five times a week can supply additional EFAs. Walnuts are an excellent source of the omega-3 EFAs, especially when they are mixed in with hazelnuts, almonds and peanuts. Seeds can also be a rich source of EFAs. Besides roasted flaxseeds, other seeds can be added to the diet as well: one tablespoon of sesame seeds contains five grams of EFA plus vitamins E, iron and zinc; one tablespoon of poppy seeds contain four grams of fat plus calcium, and iron; one tablespoon of pumpkin seeds contains twelve grams of fat plus vitamin E, iron, magnesium, potassium, zinc, selenium and fiber; one tablespoon of sunflower seeds contains fourteen grams of fat plus vitamin E, Thiamin, magnesium, iron, zinc, folic acid and fiber.

Malic Acid/Magnesium Malate

Malic acid, or magnesium malate, can be helpful in reducing pain and increasing energy production due to the fact it can reverse localized hypoxia (low muscle-tissue oxygen) in patients with chronic fibromyalgia. Studies have shown in muscle biopsies taken from affected areas in patients with FMS, the process of muscle tissue glycolysis is inhibited. *Glycolysis* is the breakdown of glucose or glycogen compounds by enzymes that produces pyruvic (lactic) acid, which then releases energy into the body.

These studies have also shown that low levels of high-energy phosphates (ATP, ADP and phosphocreatine) were found. In other words, lack of oxygen in the cells of muscle tissue (*hypoxia*) causes a marked reduction in the production and release of bio-chemical energy into the body. Furthermore, low oxygen levels in muscle tissue can contribute to muscle pain because glycolysis results in muscle tissue breakdown and mitochondrial damage. The *mitochondria* are the small round or rod-shaped bodies found inside the *cytoplasm* (a complex of chemical compounds) of most cells that produce enzymes for the metabolic conversion of food into energy.

Under aerobic conditions, the oxidation of malate into *oxalo-acetate* (acetic acid) builds up in muscle tissue to an excess level that inhibits glycolysis, which then results in hypoxia. Malic acid (magnesium malate) has the ability to "remove the accumulating reducing equivalent" (the build up of acetic acid). This allows malic acid to reverse hypoxia and its subsequent inhibition of energy production. By reversing the negative effects of hypoxia, malic acid can improve energy production in people with chronic fibromyalgia and chronic fatigue syndrome as well as maximize the energy production of healthy people as well.

A 2005 article reprinted from *Nutritional News* stated that, "Malic acid may be used as a general supplement, ensuring an optimal level of malic acid within the cells and thus maintaining an optimal level of energy production." An amount of 1200 – 2400 mg per day of malic acid was suggested from studies showing improved pain levels in patients with chronic FMS within 48 hours. The chronic constriction of muscles, ligaments and tendons in people with severe fibromyalgia may not be characterized as an aerobic exercise because there is no increase in heart rate, however the depleting effects are the same and are accumulative.

In a healthy person, the effects of an aerobic workout are temporary because when the workout ends, the body recovers and returns to normal. When muscle constriction is chronic throughout the body and the muscles remain hard at work even while sleeping, as in severe chronic FMS, the effects of overspent and fatigued muscle tissue can accumulate, resulting in ever increasing pain and weakness.

There are other hypoxia-related conditions such as chronic respiratory and circulatory insufficiencies like asthma, emphysema and diabetes that are associated with a deficiency in energy production that can benefit from this form of supplement as well. So, adding unsaturated EFAs to your diet while avoiding saturated animal fats, and adding malic acid to your protocol can go a long way in helping your body produce more energy.

Excitotoxins
Glutamate, Aspartame and Alcohol

Exitotoxins in our food are another dietary consideration that can cause adverse effects in the body. Studies have shown that excitotoxins can dramatically exacerbate chronic FMS and other pain syndrome symptoms, and that simply eliminating them from the diet can provide pain relief. Excitotoxins are molecules that act as ***"excitatory neurotransmitters"*** in the brain that lead to neurotoxicity when they are used in excess. Excitotoxins are found in substances such as aspartate (in aspartame), glutamate (in monosodium glutamate) and alcohol. These molecules have the ability to pass through the biochemical blood-brain barrier and freely enter the regions of the brain that other substances are blocked from penetrating.

Excitotoxins can pass through circumventricular organs by way of the hypothalamus, and their excitotoxic mechanism can destroy the neurons of these organs. Excitotoxins are ***excitatory amino acids*** (EAAs) and the theory is that their neurotoxic effects can interfere with the function of the hypothalamus, resulting in the disturbance of hormonal biorhythms. This disturbance can stimulate the pituitary to release the hormone cortisol and stimulate the adrenals to release the hormone adrenalin (the two "death hormones").

This in turn causes prolonged firing of peripheral nociceptive neurons that act on the dorsal horn spinal cord, which leads to chronic pain and central nervous system hypersensitization. By eliminating glutamate (MSG), aspartate (aspartame) and alcohol from the diet, the adverse neurotoxic affect of these excitotoxins on the human central nervous system can be largely avoided. I remember a rheumatologist telling me to avoid all alcohol because it is a "strong neurotoxin."

Glutamate

Glutamate in monosodium glutamate (MSG) is the sodium salt of the amino acid *"glutamic acid"* and was mistakenly declared by the U.S. Food and Drug Administration in the late 1980's as a harmless food substance, along with salt and baking powder. It is used as an additive to enhance the flavor of certain foods by stimulating glutamic acid receptors on the tongue. The symptom complex caused by MSG includes headaches, weakness, muscle tightness, numbness or tingling and flushing. Studies have shown that in addition to exacerbating chronic FMS symptoms, conditions such as asthma can also be worsened after eating foods containing MSG.

Glutamate has also been shown to destroy hypothalamic neurons in the brain. The abnormal function (excitatory effects) of glutamate receptors through the use of excess dietary glutamate has been linked to neurological disorders such as Alzheimer's disease and Huntington's chorea. Glutamate is rapidly absorbed into the bloodstream and can be found in nearly every processed food, appearing under the names monosodium glutamate, gelatin, hydrolyzed vegetable protein, textured protein and yeast extract. Watch out for it!

Aspartame

Aspartame (the excitatory amino acid aspartate) was first marketed in 1981 to be used in foods, beverages and drugs, and has become the dominant artificial sweetener of modern society. Aspartate (aspartame) is equal to glutamate in its ability to destroy hypothalamic neurons and when combined with glutamate, its neurotoxic effects are compounded. Furthermore, studies have shown aspartame to be associated with increased incidence of brain tumors in animals. Its human symptom complex includes headaches, seizures, dizziness, movement disorders, urticaria (skin rash), angioedema (angio means blood or lymph vessels; edema means an abnormal build up of fluid between tissue cells) and anaphylaxis (extreme sensitivity to a specific protein or drug).

Avoid using artificial sweeteners containing aspartame such as diet drinks, etc. and use substitutes for sugar such as Stevia or Splenda instead. These sugar substitutes are showing up more and more in products on the market place and in packets on the tables of restaurants (Splenda is the yellow stuff). Eliminate the potential of glutamate and/or aspartate to exacerbate chronic FMS symptoms via spinal cord excitation by simply avoiding dietary excitotoxins (including alcohol). This can be an effective and benign treatment option that can have noticeable results in relieving many chronic FSM symptoms. Avoiding aspartame is also a good practice for healthy people as well.

Anti-Inflammatory Protocol

Nutrition can be combined and used for specific purposes, and one important purpose in any condition that is associated with chronic pain is to reduce pain and inflammation. An anti-inflammatory nutritional protocol that is safe and effective is as follows:

Omega-3 essential fatty acids: EPA oil, DHA oil, or flaxseed oil, or fish oil daily.
Double bond antioxidants: Co-Q 10, vitamins C and E.
Ice: one to four times per day, ten to twenty minutes at a time.
Breathing exercises: In through nose for six or seven seconds, hold four seconds, out through the mouth in four seconds; four in a row, four times per day.
Increase in aerobic fitness: (if possible) Example - walking daily.
Avoid trans-fatty acids (TFAs): Avoid hydrogenated vegetable oils (margarines) that are high in pro-inflammatory omega-6 arachidonic acid.
Five to nine fresh fruits and vegetables per day.
Reduce or stop smoking.
Avoid all forms of excitotoxins: The molecules that excite neurotransmitters in the CNS, such as MSG (hydrolyzed vegetable protein), aspartame and alcohol.
Avoid or reduce red meat: High in pro-inflammatory omega-6 arachidonic acid.
Avoid caffeine: It leaches out calcium phosphates and causes tightening of tissues.

Tryptophan: Tryptophan is an essential amino acid (a part of animal proteins) that can offer a synergistic benefit known to be very calming. It gives an overall feeling of peace and well-being. Tryptophan is found in foods that are readily available in the average daily diet. These foods are: apples, bananas, milk, turkey and low sugar/low fat chocolate (70% + dark chocolate). Turkey not only contains high levels of tryptophan, it also contains proteins and multiple complex vitamins that induce a peaceful, sleepy feeling. Aside from offering a feeling of calmness, tryptophan also offers pain relief.

Foods high in this essential amino acid stimulate the production and release of biochemical neurotransmitter serotonin in the brain. The stimulation of serotonin production initiates a neurotransmitter cascade involving endogenous opiates (neurotransmitters associated with pain relief), GABA (neurotransmitters associated with minor tranquilizers) and dopamine (the neurotransmitter of euphoria). The result of tryptophan stimulating the increased production and release of serotonin is a measure of pain relief accompanied by a feeling of relaxation and euphoria.

Another component of the synergism of tryptophan is sugar. The action of sugar in the system begins the above mentioned neurotransmitter cascade by increasing serotonin in the synapses (the junctions between nerve cells where they almost meet and where they transmit signals). Sugar does this by creating an elevation of insulin, which knocks other competing amino acids (organic acids) out of the bloodstream and consequently allows the amino acid tryptophan immediate and exclusive passage into the brain. There it combines with tryptophan-hydroxylace, a decomposing and reducing agent that acts in the synthesis of organic molecules to synthesize serotonin.

Since serotonin production is "rate-related" to the amount of tryptophan available and the serotonin synthesizing neurons in the brain, the more tryptophan that is consumed, the more serotonin will be synthesized. When serotonin levels drop, food cravings begin. In addition, studies have shown the use of a complex of serotonin and histamine, along with their precursors L-tryptophan and L-histidine, has resulted in an increase in resistance toward hypoxia (low levels of oxygen in tissue) in mice and rats. So, eat plenty of foods high in tryptophan, and follow that turkey sandwich at lunch or a hot slice of turkey at dinner with an apple, a banana, a scoop of low-fat chocolate ice cream or a small piece of dark chocolate, and that should do the trick.

Dietary tryptophan has another benefit for the body because it is the essential amino acid responsible for the body's own production of vitamins B-1 and B-5 (Niacin). As a general rule, the human body cannot manufacture vitamins, and what we get comes from our food plus whatever we add through nutrition supplementation. However, niacin (B-5) is different from other vitamins because it can be synthesized from trypto-phan. Rich food sources for niacin and tryptophan include red meats, poultry, fish, liver, kidneys, eggs, nuts, brewer's yeast and wheat germ.

The recommended daily allowance for niacin is between 15 and 20 mg per day, however a therapeutic dose, that is niacin in larger amounts, is roughly 500 mg two or three times a day for treatment of high serum (blood) cholesterol. Using "no-flush" or "flush-free" niacin will avoid the dreaded niacin flush and other side effects of regular niacin. Even time-release prescription niacin can cause a minor intermittent flushing to occur with each timed release over a twenty-four hour period.

A niacin flush can last up to an hour and can be very uncomfortable, even painful for someone with chronic FMS. Another benefit of niacin (niacinamide/B5) is an increase in circulation throughout the body, espe-cially to our extremities like fingers and toes that are characteristically cold due to poor circulation related to conditions like diabetes or from the chronic constriction of soft tissues in FMS. When you are taking niacin as apart of your daily nutritional protocol you may notice that you are warmer and pinker.

The Glycemic Index

The Glycemic Index (GI) of food is an index that ranks foods on how they specifically affect blood sugar levels in comparison to pure glucose. The GI is used primarily to evaluate the metabolism of carbohydrates. Protein and fat do not cause blood sugar level to rise very much, except when they are combined with carbohydrates that rank high on the Glyce-mic Index. The original GI sets glucose (sugar) at 100, although it is now more common in the U.S. to see white bread set at 100. Glucose is a sim-ple sugar produced in plants through photosynthesis and in animals by the conversion of carbohydrates combined with proteins and fats.

Fructose is a sugar found in certain fruits and in honey. Although glucose and fructose (starches and sugars) are both carbohydrates, foods lowest on the GI do not raise blood sugar significantly. Consequently, they release far less insulin than foods high on the scale. The fact "not all carbohydrates are created equal" is used in the formation of the hypogly-cemic diet that controls blood sugar levels for people with low blood sug-ar.

The hypoglycemic dietary guideline simply states people with hypo-glycemia can eat all they want of foods low on the GI, moderate amounts of foods in the mid-range, and must avoid foods at the top of the scale. Beginning at the top of the GI, the food-glucose values of twenty com-mon foods are listed as follows:

Glucose	100
Grapes	100
Baked russet potato	98
Carrots	92
Honey	87
Cornflakes	80
Wheat bread	72
White rice	72
White bread	69
Brown rice	66
Sweet corn	59
Sucrose	59
Peas	53
Pasta	45-50
Apples	39
Tomatoes	38
Milk	34
Yogurt	34
Peaches	26
Fructose	25

To convert the above index into the white-bread scale, you simply multiply the values by 0.7 to get the exact measurements, however the relative relationships between glucose conversion and food will remain the same. Because foods vary greatly in their ability to release insulin, a potato for instance (98 on the scale) – gram weight per gram weight – cannot be substituted for an apple (39 on the scale).

Aside from the hypoglycemic diet, most of the popular low carbohydrate diets are designed for weight loss and for lowering serum cholesterol and are not geared toward controlling blood sugar levels. These diets commonly remove all white foods from the diet, such as white bread, pasta, white rice, potatoes and sugar. Also, diets that are simply based on caloric restriction do not take into consideration the glycemic index.

Studies have shown people with chronic FMS feel better overall when they follow a hypoglycemic diet guideline and keep their blood sugar levels even by avoiding spikes in blood sugar caused by eating foods high on the glycemic index. Keep in mind there are two types of carbohydrates: 1) simple carbohydrates - sugars including table sugar (sucrose), fruit sugar (fructose), honey (maltose), and milk sugar (lactose) and 2) complex carbohydrates including starches such as bread, pasta, rice, potatoes, cereals, peas and legumes (beans). When carbohydrates are ingested, the pancreas responds by producing and releasing insulin, a hormone that clears excess glucose from the bloodstream.

The higher the carbohydrate is on the glycemic index, the more glucose is converted and released into the bloodstream, and the more insulin is produced to clear out the excess. Insulin clears out excess glucose (energy/calories) from the blood by directing it into muscles and fat cells of the body for storage in the form of glycogen, along with amino acids which are the building blocks of protein and fat. This is why **insulin** is called "the storage hormone." When the storage capacities of muscle and fat cells reach their maximums, the remaining glucose is then converted into fatty acids that turn into what we call unwanted body fat cells or triglycerides (surplus energy stored as fat).

People with chronic FMS crave carbohydrates and sugar in a futile attempt to gain more energy due to their chronic fatigue and dysenergism. According to Dr. Paul St. Amand in his book "*What your Doctor May Not Tell You About Fibromyalgia,*" 40% of women and 20% of men with FMS also have hypoglycemia (carbohydrate intolerance). In addition, giving in to sugar and heavy starch cravings (simple and complex carbohydrates) for energy will eventually lead to hypoglycemia in patients with chronic FMS who did not have it originally.

These cravings will begin to dissipate after you have been on a hypoglycemic diet for a couple weeks and should be gone in one or two months. The reason giving in to these cravings causes hypoglycemia (low blood sugar) is because when you eat high amounts of sugars and starches, your pancreas pumps proportional amounts of insulin into the blood in spikes to clear out the excess glucose from the blood and drives it into muscle and fat cells, resulting in low blood sugar levels.

Along with the glucose, phosphate ions are also driven into the cells because one of their jobs is to attach themselves to glucose molecules inside the cell. Combining sugars and starches with caffeine makes it worse because caffeine prolongs the action of insulin. Therefore, repeat surges of insulin into the body eventually leads to hypoglycemia which adds its own set of symptoms to those of chronic FMS, and this makes for an even more miserable combination.

Furthermore, insulin signals appropriate kidney cells to reabsorb phosphate ions that should have been filtered from the blood and eliminated in the urine, and re-circulates them back into the bloodstream and into many cells in the body. Since muscle cells are most responsive to the instruction of insulin to absorb large amounts of phosphate ions, these are the cells most affected by this specific insulin directive in FMS patients. The result is an excess of phosphate ions in the muscle cells.

The science of physiology and biochemistry has shown the presence of excess phosphate ions in the part of the cell called the mitochondria (the cell matrix where APT/energy is produced) will slow down and even block energy production.

The cells highest in their activity requiring the most energy (like the brain and the muscles) will be the first to be affected by lack of energy, thus the muscle pain, weakness and "fibro-fog" of chronic FMS.

In addition, where there is an excess of phosphate ions there is also an excess of calcium molecules. Phosphate ions carry two negative charges to maintain the bioelectrical equilibrium inside the cells. Calcium molecules carry two positive charges (agents) to serve as the main buffer for phosphates, and are also used to "call a muscle cell to action" when the muscle is stimulated by the brain or an outside stimulus. We all know what happens when opposites attract, there is no separating them. They marry for better or for worse and the rest is history.

Furthermore, a calcium molecule is like a battery terminal that stores up these little agents (positive charges) until they are needed and temporarily releases them when they are. This store and release function requires energy to perform, and when ATP production is slowed or blocked in the cell matrix from the presence of excess phosphate ions, the energy needed to stop the calcium molecule from engaging in its "call to action" in the muscle cell after a stimulus has ended, is not there.

The result is the calcium molecule with its two positive charges is allowed to sit for too long a time inside muscle tissue affected by this metabolic error. Consequently, the muscle is subjected to being continually called into action and overworked to a point of exhaustion, fatigue, weakness and chronic pain. There is a popular theory that the primary cause of chronic FMS is a genetic kidney malfunction causing the recirculation of excess phosphate ions back into the bloodstream creating the above metabolic error. The moral of this story is if you have chronic FMS, you simply must choose to eat correctly. If you give into your cravings for sugar and fast carbohydrates, your body will release large amounts of insulin in spikes that will drive more phosphate ions with its disgruntled partner calcium into your tissue cells.

When this occurs, you will likely feel even worse after you indulge, and not better. Keep in mind that the demand for ATP (energy) production is so high in people with chronic FMS that this craving is naturally going to be very difficult to resist. However it may help if you understand why no amount of sugar or carbohydrates can satisfy the demand for energy in a fibromyalgic. Your energy simply must come from eating the proper foods, supplementing your diet with the proper nutritional supplements, frequent rests during the day, practicing deep breathing twice a day and restorative sleep at night.

As I mentioned early in the chapter on physical theories of cause, the presence of excess phosphates has been found when testing the muscle tissue of people with FMS, and is the only test that can visibly indicate a possible FMS diagnosis.

However, whether or not a kidney malfunction resulting in this finding is due to a genetic tendency that has somehow been triggered, or if a malfunction of the kidneys is simply due to another bizarre metabolic malfunction in the widespread mayhem of symptoms manifested under the umbrella of chronic fibromyalgia, the bottom line is that excess phosphates have been found in the tissue of a fibromyalgic person.

Bingeing on sugars and starches (carbohydrates) for energy causes your insulin to spike and high levels of insulin drive even more phosphates into your muscle tissues, these excess phosphates do unwillingly couple with excess calcium molecules and ultimately make you feel worse, not better. The good news is it does not take long to lose your cravings and begin to feel better on the proper nutritional protocol. Personally, I happen to believe that problems with the kidneys or any other system in the body are all part of the wide range of FMS symptoms, and is simply another symptom being mistaken for the cause.

Cholesterol Lowering Diet

Complimentary to a hypoglycemic diet for the purpose of feeling better and being healthier is a cholesterol lowering diet. A hypoglycemic diet generally involves avoiding foods high on the glycemic index, eating a moderate amount of foods in the medium range of the index and all you want of foods low on the index. A cholesterol lowering diet usually suggests reducing saturated fat (the biggest culprit, mostly from animal products) and full-fat dairy products, avoiding refined sugars and carbohydrates, eating lots of vegetables and some fruits, and eating only lean meats and fish. It also includes whole grains cereals and rye or dark breads. My osteopath said to take white foods out of the diet, eat lots of fresh, dark colored foods and lean meat, chicken and fish.

Both diets support cooking with canola or olive oil, eating omelets made from egg whites or Egg Beaters and sugar-free turkey. The two guidelines are not only beneficial for people with fibromyalgia, they would make anyone feel better and be healthier. Avoiding triggering hypoglycemia and lowering serum (blood) cholesterol levels is especially important for someone with chronic FMS because with all the misery they already suffer from, adding these two enemies to the fight is much more than adding insult to injury. The problems high cholesterol alone can bring to the arena, such as cardiovascular diseases and arteriosclerosis, are a horrific way to compound the array of usual FMS symptoms and these problems do not need to be provoked.

Three types of cholesterol
directly impacting your health

1) *Low-density lipoprotein* (LDL) is the bad cholesterol. LDL is responsible for most of the damage done by cholesterol in the arteries, such as accumulating on the walls (hardening of the arteries) and constricting and even blocking the flow of blood. The higher level of LDL you have in your blood, the greater your risk of disease. The healthy range for LDL on a lipid blood panel test is 50 – 129.

2) *High-density lipoprotein* (HDL) is the good cholesterol. It works to balance LDL in the blood. It does this by literally picking up LDL cholesterol in the blood and transporting it back to the liver, which works to eliminate it from the body. By doing this, HDL helps prevent cholesterol from building up on the walls of the arteries, and helps prevent heart disease. And guess what? Omega-3 EFAs help the production of more HDL! The healthy range for HDL on a lipid blood panel is 30 – 85.

3) *Triglycerides* are neither good not bad, are a form of fatty acid carried through the bloodstream making up the bulk of what is stored in soft tissue as unwanted body fat. The presence of triglycerides in the blood is normally found to be minimal, however when triglyceride levels prove high, it means the lipoproteins containing the cholesterol contributing to coronary artery disease (CAD) is also high. The healthy range for triglycerides on a lipid blood panel is 0 – 200.

The healthy range for the total of all three types of cholesterol together is 120 – 200. Within this range however, it is important that the HDL is in the higher range of normal, especially if the LDL is high. Serum cholesterol levels in the blood are affected by genetic heredity (how fast your body creates LDL cholesterol in the liver, and how fast the body eliminates it) and by the food you eat with regard to its cholesterol content. Interestingly, since the liver manufactures all the cholesterol most people will ever need, you do not need to add cholesterol to your diet.

In addition, following the cholesterol diet guidelines and combining it with exercise will not only help bring down your cholesterol, it will also be a natural way to lose weight. Excess body fat increases LDL cholesterol, and the single act of losing weight may be all you need to lower your cholesterol to safe levels if it proves to be too high. In addition, physical exercise tends to raise HDL levels that consequently lower the LDL level in the blood. Adding specific nutritional supplements is another effective way to help lower your total cholesterol.

For instance, antioxidants such as vitamin C (2000 – 5000 mg daily) and vitamin E (400 – 800 IU daily) have been proven to inhibit and slow the development of cholesterol oxidation onto the walls of arteries. Fish oil or flaxseed oil containing omega-3 fatty acids (6000 – 8000 mg once or twice daily) have been shown to reduce high levels of triglycerides by an average of 35%.

Niacin (vitamin B5 – found in wheat, meat and dairy) taken in doses well above daily requirement (1500–3000 mg daily – the flush free kind as a therapeutic dose) can lower your total cholesterol profile because nicotinic acid lowers LDL and triglycerides while at the same time raises HDL – the good cholesterol that helps remove the bad cholesterol from the blood. Studies have shown that inositol hexanicotinate (flush-free niacin) "appears to have the greatest potential to increase HDL cholesterol by 30%."

In addition to vitamins C and E, omega-3 fatty acid and niacin, there are other nutritional supplements that offer synergistic benefits in addition to dietary modifications that can be very effective in elevating HDL cholesterol and reducing total serum cholesterol, thereby reducing the associated risk.

Additional cholesterol lowering nutrients are:
Artichoke leaf extract – 300 mg three times daily
Curcumin (turmeric root) – 900 to 1800 mg daily
Garlic – 900 to 8000 mg daily in liquid extract (most important of these)
Green tea (95% polyphenol extract) – 350 mg daily
Gugulipid (made from the resin of the Commiphora Mukul tree of northern-central India) – 140 mg one or two times daily
Selenium – 200 to 600 mcg daily
Soy Protein Extract – two heaping teaspoons (five to six grams or 5000 to 6000 mg) of powder daily, or one capsule of Mega Soy Extract - 135 mg/40% extract twice daily.

Adding what you can to your daily protocol of diet plus the right amount of nutritional supplements plus exercise of one kind or another, may be all you need to get high cholesterol under control without having to take a drug that will tax your liver. These drugs have side effects like pain and weakness in the legs, issue warnings to people with liver problems, and do not always work well with other drugs you may be taking.

Your doctor can advise you on these points, and periodic cholesterol evaluations (every three months or so) can tell you if your diet and nutritional protocol plus exercise is working for you.

Diet, exercise and genetics are all factors in serum cholesterol, and it makes sense to address the problem with natural alternatives first before trying a drug.

Bear in mind that medical schools do not offer doctors extensive training in nutrition. What additional knowledge they acquire must be attained on their own, either through research articles in nutritional journals, seminars or books. This may be difficult for them to do because after medical school they must immediately begin practicing medicine in order to pay for the enormous cost of their education. In addition, if they open their own practice, they must subsidize the costs of overhead expenditures such as employee wages, social security and workers' compensation insurance; operating expenses such as office and medical supplies and equipment; overhead expenses such as rent, heating, water and electricity; and finally the extreme cost of medical malpractice insurance.

They must foot all these expenses and make a decent living as well and the pressure can be enormous. Furthermore, when their practice is built up to full capacity their time is more limited than ever. It takes a very dedicated physician to devote personal time on continued self-education in areas outside their orthodox medical training, such as nutrition and alternative medicine. I admire the ones who do.

The arena of alternative medicine is largely an unknown mystery for the majority of practicing physicians, and can be seen by them in the light of their orthodox medical training as being somewhat of a myth. I suggest you find a physician that not only knows about chronic fibromyalgia, but also knows something about therapeutic nutritional protocols and alternative therapies that can be helpful to you. If their focus is primarily set on matching symptoms with a diagnosis and giving drugs they are trained to use to "manage the condition" and are not open to alternatives, they may not be the right doctors for you.

You can also try providing your doctor with information and articles for their perusal on therapeutic nutrition and alternative therapies you are trying, and give them feedback on how these therapies work or do not work for you. A conscientious physician will appreciate your sharingthis kind of information with them, especially when they may not otherwise have the opportunity to acquire it, and will be happy to work with you in your efforts to improve your condition without pushing the standard drug protocols used today to manage chronic FMS symptoms.

Most importantly, make sure your doctor knows that many of the current beliefs about chronic FMS are not necessarily true, such as: the etiology (cause) is unknown; the condition has no cure; the condition is always degenerative; and the only hope to improve future quality of life is to manage symptoms with heavy prescription drugs. The reality is none of these beliefs are true.

I understand the medical profession would not be privy yet to the cause of FMS because it lies outside their area of expertise, however I would like to ask one question here. If the cause of chronic FMS is currently unknown amongst the medical profession, how can they possibly say to anyone with any degree of certainty that this condition has no cure simply because their current methods of treatment are not working to cure it? Why not simply say that there is currently no known effective treatment or cure for chronic FMS in their own arena of orthodox medicine, and the best thing to do is keep looking in other arenas?

- 1995 -
Valerie Lumley (Co-existing condition caus-ing neurological disorder.) 5-22-97 Sent

cc: Jeff Lester, DC
cc: Larry Petersen,
I DO
cc: Karen Cohen,
06-26-02 DC
6905 cc: D. Kirby, DC

Re: Injury 11-14-93, Doing ONE crunch/situp with hands behind neck from R. elbow to L. knee. point A. Felt a mild pop₃ & pain on R. side at point B. neck

Then; For 2½ years;

"R.C. (Atlas Occipital) joint + C-1 (Atlas)"

→ Pt. A

→ Difficult turning head to L., & pain!

→ Burning pain & acute spasm.

→ Spasms & pain.

→ Point B.

"Constant" is true in every "flair-up" & entensifies acutely at point A.

● = Central areas of pain = "CONSTANT"

Q. Why this constant? (asked repeatedly)

A. "Don't try to pinpoint pain. It will move around like a butterfly."

A. Maybe because I am R. handed.

A. One side is weaker than other.

A. Several other non-specifics A.'s.

A. The weakest link.

Points:

1) All other pain has come & gone & moved around, except for "constant."

2) The only time "Constant" dissipated was when I was taking pain killers & receiving osteo-pathic treatment once or twice a week in combination with nortryplene.

(over)

Hollister

3) The only person who has given this specific attention is <u>Dr. Brandon</u> in Hollister who said that because of the way we are wired, the nerves that are irritated at point A. are manifested in pain at point B. ∴ His suggestion was osteopathy and a manual adjustment at the top of the neck (the later I chose to hold in reserve). He feels problem is at the top of the neck, and the cause.

FACTS ABOUT PT. A; (@ top of the neck)
1) Where I was hit by semi-truck front bumper sustaining an open wound, mild concussion & whip-lash to L. 25 yrs. ago.
2) Where I landed at approx. age 6 when I fell off of a 5' retaining wall.
3) The location of acute pain during my "flair-ups".
4) Near TMJ trouble on R. jaw.
5) Where migrains seem to begin during PMS monthly.
6) I have always slept on R. side.
7) All my chronic pain is on R. side.

The Atlas
Subluxation

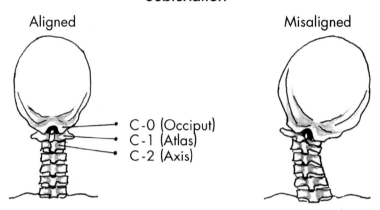

Aligned

Misaligned

- C-0 (Occiput)
- C-1 (Atlas)
- C-2 (Axis)

The Atlas (C-1) must be precisely aligned with the Occiput (C-2) above the Axis (C-2) below in order for the brain's life-giving and healing signals to be delivered into the body through the spinal cord and central nervous system undistorted. Even the slightest misalignment of the Atlas will cause a kink in the spinal cord at the foramen magnum that results in 1) pinching of the brainstem where it meets the spinal cord 2) tugging and spasms of the muscles of the neck that pinch the cervical nerves and blood vessels traveling to and from the brain 3) distortion of brain signals into and from the body 4) torque on the entire meninges, causing the great nerve trunks to over-fire at their attachments up and down the spine, and 5) a chronic brainstem injury that causes the entire central nervous system to become hyperactive and hypersensitive. These combined effects create the body-wide system and malfunctions in chronic fibromyalgia syndrome. Aligning the Atlas and subsequent compensatory subluxation and cervical myopathy that this misalignment creates, combined with rehabilitating the body, a nutrition and diet protocol, homeopathy, and reducing stress through essential lifestyle changes, will cure this condition.

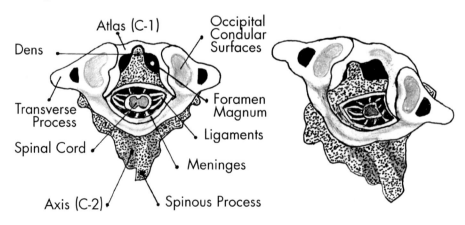

Atlas (C-1)

Dens

Occipital Condular Surfaces

Transverse Process

Foramen Magnum

Spinal Cord

Ligaments

Meninges

Axis (C-2)

Spinous Process

Effects of the Atlas Subluxation
Tight and Spasmed Muscle Groups

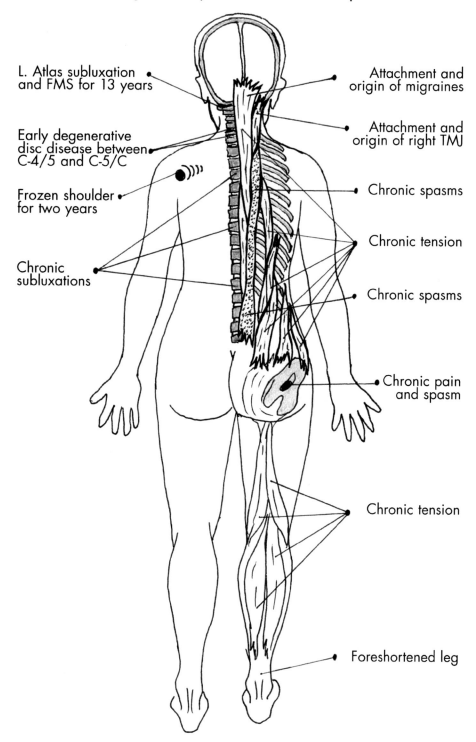

L. Atlas subluxation and FMS for 13 years

Early degenerative disc disease between C-4/5 and C-5/C

Frozen shoulder for two years

Chronic subluxations

Attachment and origin of migraines

Attachment and origin of right TMJ

Chronic spasms

Chronic tension

Chronic spasms

Chronic pain and spasm

Chronic tension

Foreshortened leg

To Live Deliberately

We must learn to awaken and keep ourselves awake by an infinite expectation of the dawn, which does not forsake us in our soundest sleep;

For we are encouraged that humans can elevate their lives by their own conscious endeavor.

It is something to be able to paint a picture, or to carve a statue, and so to make a few objects beautiful;

But it is far more glorious to carve and paint the very atmosphere and medium through which we look, which morally we can do.

To affect the quality of the day, that is the highest of arts.

It is the task of every person to make his or her life the most elevated and critical hour.

Why should we live in such a hurry and waste of life? I wish to live deliberately.

I wish to learn what life has to teach, and not, when I come to die, discover that I have not lived.

Nor do I wish to practice resignation. I wish to live deep and suck out the marrow of life. If it proves to be mean, then to get the whole genuine meanness of it, and publish its meanness to the whole world.

Or if it is sublime, to know it by experience, and to be able to give a true account of it.

Henry D. Thoreau

Chapter Eight
Discovering the Cure

For the fibromyalgic, the pathway to a lasting cure is littered with assumptions, beliefs and theories about FMS that are outdated, misplaced and misdirected from the scientific community, the medical profession and others who do not have it. The job of the fibromyalgic is to continue on the healing path and step over the obstacles that might otherwise deter them. One of the beliefs that may lie cross your path is that you brought this illness on yourself through unresolved psychological issues or unfinished business. Here is where the issue of Karma enters into the equation and is important for the FMS patient to understand what Karma really is if they are going to dodge the bullets of extreme guilt and hopelessness and the stress these factors cause.

The Law of Karma maintains there is no good act without divine will or the grace of God and that every deliberate action has its own consequence that pursues the doer, often beyond the grave (unfinished business). The question of Karmic debt has been raised to me repeatedly during my quest to discover the cure for chronic fibromyalgia. Searching for answers to possible causes for chronic FMS is naturally accompanied by such spiritual questions as "Why is this happening to me?" and "What have I done to deserve this?"

The first aspect of Karma is that it is individual, meaning each person instigates or creates his or her own specific Karma and everyone has different Karma that is not due to, nor is it caused by, anyone else. The law of Karma in the spiritual universe is similar to Newton's Mechanical Law in the physical universe which states, "For each action, there is an equal and opposite reaction." This means in spiritual terms that as you do, so will be done to you, and as you sew, so shall you reap.

To understand Karma is to understand that nobody gets away with anything in this dimension. However the power of grace can help absolve a tremendous amount of Karmic debt. Grace can be manifested through forgiveness and meditation that brings with it enlightenment (understanding of what has and is now occurring). As our souls grow

227

and evolve through karmic lessons we aspire toward spiritual perfection and a total lack of selfishness, obsession and egoic mind.

I feel that in addition to cause and effect, there is also what I call the "law of random occurrences" which simply means that sometimes things can happen by accident or just because they do, and that not everything carries with it a hidden karmic meaning. Sometimes a cigar is just a cigar. The notion that everything that happens in this dimension carries with it Karmic meaning can become an unnecessary source of stress.

When a person suffers a random accidental injury to the neck, such as whiplash from an automobile accident or a blow to the head from a fall that causes chronic FMS, this does not mean they brought this onto themselves as some kind of karmic payback for something they have done. And just because they happen to be experiencing the pressure of some form of Karmic lesson in their life (which I believe most people are) in addition to a random accidental occurrence does not mean that the two are related. Both things can very easily occur separately at the same time, and are therefore mutually exclusive coincidences.

The best way I can illustrate that being stricken with chronic FMS does not mean that you have done something horrible is to tell my story; how I discovered the cause and the cure to chronic fibromyalgia that empowered me to take my life back. Be assured that I have created plenty of my own Karma in this lifetime from consequences of choices I made that were both wise and unwise, but I have always sought to face life head on, hungry to learn my lessons along the way. I am the first to admit that when I was younger I had to experience things more than once before I became enlightened enough by their messages to apply what I learned to my life and make better choices. This is simply an example of the average human being hard at work on the painful path of spiritual evolution toward enlightenment.

Chronic FMS constitutes a challenge that is nearly insurmountable to the average person. Experiencing chronic FMS in addition to my personal Karma was truly an intense combination of challenges. The only part of these challenges that I can say was not part of my personal Karma was the cervical spine injury that triggered chronic FMS and the subsequent effects and losses.

I was very fortunate to have married a man who was loyal and devoted, who did not run out the door when I became ill and who supported me as I searched for the cause and cure for this condition. Also, I never stopped believing in the premise that no matter what is going on in a person's life, one must always keep moving forward through whatever is happening with a fierce refusal to resign or become complacent no matter how difficult or how slow going it may be. This is the only way through and out of any unacceptable situation. So, one day at a time I continued to move forward and never, ever accepted this situation as permanent no matter what I was told by one medical care provider after another.

Deep down I always knew I would find a way out of chronic FMS as long as I kept searching, hoping and believing in myself and in the power of choice. I knew I was capable of guiding myself because I had been doing it since I was a small child. I simply had to choose to trust my intuition, listen to my quiet inner voice of reason, take charge of my condition and my life and choose to make the tough, necessary life-changes that would make it possible to defeat the overpowering monster that wanted to devoured me.

After suffering for many years with no real help from anyone, I realized that getting well was going to be up to me, and that I was going to have to leave the care of the medical profession and look for help elsewhere. I decided to become fiercely proactive. Considering the possibility of existing, suffering and declining with chronic FMS for the rest of your life, I believed that no matter how difficult it might become, choosing what works to cure FMS would be far easier than the alternative.

There is an old axiom called "Akums Razor" which states, "When all things are equal, the simplest explanation must be the truth." This axiom addresses the cause in that when you look at all the complex theories of cause out there, some are widely known while others are remote and even seem a bit wacky. The notion of a simple Atlas kink subluxation (misaligned C-1 vertebra) and the resulting brainstem injury, cervical myopathy, compensative spinal subluxations, and subsequent body imbalances being the cause of chronic FMS may seem most perplexing in its simplicity. However something as soundly and profoundly simple as a misalignment of the Atlas does in fact account for all of the crazy symptoms of chronic FMS, and therefore must be the truth. Where is it written that something as complex as chronic FMS must have an equally complex cause?

Another old axiom that states, "When all other contingencies fail, that which remains, however improbable it may seem, must be the truth." This axiom addresses the cure in that when you look at all of the "management therapies" and "treatment protocols" that have been used by conventional medicine with little or no success, the re-alignment of a misaligned Atlas vertebra and subsequent spinal subluxations and the rehabilitation of the body, may seem an improbable cure for the long list of FMS symptoms. However, it is the one treatment that works to alleviate all of the FMS symptoms, and therefore must be the truth. These axioms are both profoundly applicable and helpful in isolating the cause and the cure for FMS. They speak to the sublime revelations that come from good-old human common sense.

My Story

Dr. Martin Luther King, Jr. said, "Our lives begin to end the day we become silent about things that matter." It is in this spirit that I tell my true story and how I discovered the cause and cure for the chronic illness that broke in like a thief in the night and made off with my life. My story begins by accurately recounting the series of compounding injuries to my neck throughout my life and the final last-straw injury that triggered full-blown chronic FMS.

The first neck injury I can recall was when I was five or six years old walking along the top of a four-foot retaining wall behind my Grandmother's house one summer. I lost my footing and fell off the wall and landed on my head on a cement patio. I do not think I was knocked unconscious, however I remember the scorching hot cement burning my arms and legs, and that I was able to get up and go inside. I had a large goose egg on the top of my head but do not remember any other ill effects. I am not even sure I told anyone because I do not remember any adult intervention. Because children bounce back from things so well unless something is broken, I wonder if this should even be considered ground zero for the series of compounding injuries that followed throughout my life. However it is a fact, and is worth considering.

The second neck injury I can recall was when I was bucked off a horse in my early teens, landing back on my tailbone, causing whiplash to my neck and knocking the wind out of me. As I lay on the ground trying to recover my breath, I do remember severe pain both at the bottom of my spine and at the top. My step-grandfather, who owned and operated the riding stables in Carmel, California where I rode, came barreling out to the pasture where the accident occurred in his pick-up truck as soon as my horse ran back into the stables without me. I was not able to walk just yet so he and a cousin lifted me into the back of the pick-up where I could lie down and took me back to the stables. I do not remember being examined by a doctor or any further adult intervention beyond that point, but I do remember having to sit on a donut pillow for about three months and having a very stiff neck for a while. I feel this accident is well worth considering as one of the compounding injuries to my neck and spine that eventually lead to chronic FMS.

The third neck injury I can recall was when I was involved in a serious auto accident where I sustained a blow to the right side of the back of my head, splitting open my scalp and knocking me out. I was taken by ambulance to a nearby hospital, sewn up and released without so much as a thorough examination or an x-ray. I am absolutely sure this blow on the head along with the whiplash is a key injury in a compounding series of head and neck injuries. I now consider this accident to be ground zero for the kind of injury that could affectively misalignment the Atlas vertebra and cause FMS.

I do not feel this probable Atlas misalignment that would have occurred to the left and forward, was moved far enough out to trigger full-blown FMS at that time. However, when I look at my medical history of physical problems along with the life stressors that made them worse, I can see a pattern of aggravated symptoms that could very well have resulted from a hyper-sensitized central nervous system caused by this major injury to my head and neck. Because I was a strong, young person with a high tolerance to pain, my youthful vitality was able to compensate for the effects of what I now consider to be early mild-FMS and I was able to move forward with my life in spite of my physical difficulties.

The fourth neck injury I recall came sadly from a number of blows to the head delivered by my first husband. Three of these were particularly severe; one blow bounced the right side of my head off a wall and another put a front tooth through my upper lip. A third happened after I was thrown down a flight of stairs and then kicked in the head and stomach as I lay on the floor. I have to consider these because they each caused whiplash and effects such as a stiff neck, dizziness, headaches and nausea for some time afterward.

Recalling this is very unpleasant, however these occurrences cannot be discounted in the series of compounding injuries to my neck throughout my life. I was in my early to mid-twenties when these injuries occurred and still vital enough energetically to physically compensate for them, however it was becoming more and more difficult to function in life with all its stressors as time went by. After my divorce at age twenty-seven I was able to develop, create and establish a new kind of service business in the field of independent medical insurance billing while I studied music, voice and vocal performance, and traveled throughout the world to recover.

Although I was able to work full-time, I remember minor indications of mild-FMS symptoms such as pain and difficulty in lifting my left arm over my head with pull-over clothing and right side back strain that would occur from time to time, both symptoms having no apparent reason. There were many other physical indications that were more pronounced, such as a chronic hyper-acidic stomach, a foreshortened right leg for which I was prescribed a lifted shoe, right hip difficulty, right side

TMJ and female disorders that are all part of the FMS scenario. All of these were naturally exacerbated by negative life stress like any other condition is.

I think back now and marvel at the willpower I possessed to make something of myself in spite of my childhood and all the other challenges I had experienced so far. I was unaware there was such a thing as an underlying physical problem as simple as a misalignment at the top of my neck that was enough to compromise me, but not enough to disable me. It was my nature to face life head on, forge ahead and keep my focus on a goal in mind at all times. My motto has always been, "Life belongs to the tenacious."

It was not until my fifth and minor "last straw" neck injury in this series of injuries that quickly triggered full-blown, chronic FMS. This injury was insidious and covert in its simplicity, as is often the case in triggering chronic FMS. On November 14, 1993 I injured my neck while on the floor doing sit-up crunches to improve my diaphragm strength for singing. I had my hands behind my head and was pulling on my head and neck (which I did not know at the time was a strict taboo) and crunching my right elbow to my left knee. Suddenly I felt the left side of the top of my neck pop slightly and a sharp pain shoot down my back on the right side.

I felt like there was something very wrong and immediately stopped what I was doing. I lay back on the floor to rest a while but could not get comfortable, so I got up and went to rest in bed. For the next ten days I felt stiff all over and the right side of my back became more and more contracted. Then, ten days after the neck injury, I fell to the floor in extreme back pain and spasms lasting in such a way I could not get up for several hours. I had to be helped into bed, and could not move a muscle for another fourteen hours. I was taken to a Doctors on Duty office, diagnosed with muscle strain, given prescriptions for a heavy muscle relaxer, painkiller and anti-inflammatory and an order for six weeks of physical therapy. In spite of this course of treatment, my condition continued to worsen and I continued to be in so much pain that I could not sleep.

Albert Einstein said, "Ethics are a specific human concern without any greater power behind it." The key ethic of the "Hippocratic Oath" that all doctor's pledge before they graduate is, "First do no harm." This is a paradox when you consider that physicians are "practicing" medicine and you are a high paying test subject. With all their good intentions, because of the limited nature of their training they can "miss the medical boat" so easily in so many ways. After this first misdiagnosis, I "plugged into" my higher power and decided to seek help from the chiropractic profession. I drew up my analysis of what I felt could be the cause of my illness (an auto accident with a blow to the head many years ago, plus the recent injury at home) in the form of a diagram with some key questions, and I made several copies and gave one to the chiropractor.

On December 10, 1993 I saw my first chiropractor and sadly, he completely missed the mark. He took full front and side x-rays of my neck and spine and said there was a subluxation (a partial dislocation of bones that leaves them misaligned) in the fourth thoracic vertebra (T-4) that he felt was the cause, was simply of all my symptoms. When I asked him about my analysis of what might be the root cause, he said he preferred to go with only what **he** could see in the x-rays. When I looked at the x-rays, I saw nothing but perfect alignment of the thoracic area, and when I questioned his analysis he drew a circle on one of the x-rays with his pen and said, "This point on the x-ray is so minute it requires a trained eye to see it." Because he did not see the misalignment of my Atlas with his x-rays, did not notice my neck was angled to the left and my head was tilted to the right, he could not understand that what he felt was the cause simply the result of compensation stress coming from the top of my neck.

He then began a treatment plan of adjusting my spine from top to bottom three to four times a week for eight weeks with no attention to my neck. It was like bailing water out of a small, sinking boat without looking to find the hole and fix it. When my condition continued to worsen, he put me on the adjustment table face down and said, "Let out all your air and I'm going to push down really hard to make it stay in this time." He was referring to that pesky T-4 vertebra that just would not "stay in" after his adjustments and was theoretically preventing me from getting well. He leaned his body over me and pushed down so hard I felt a deep crack in my upper back between my shoulder blades and saw stars. I went back a few more times because I was still in a great deal of pain, could not sleep, could not even rest comfortably and still had to spend a lot of time in bed during the day. On February 9, 1994 after eight weeks, I left his care.

On February 10, 1994 I went to see a second chiropractor. Someone who worked in the first chiropractor's office who was very concerned about the way I was being treated recommended I seek another opinion. A friend told me about her own chiropractor who was very gentle and used a very different way of adjusting. This new doctor said she followed the methods of a French chiropractor by the name of Major Dejeuner who used pillows and wedges underneath a patient in strategic places along with deep breaths and a light touch to adjust them gently without any violence to the spine. She diagnosed me as having "an inversion in my spine from T-3 through T-6 that was pushed in so far you could set a tea cup in there."

After she adjusted me she told me to go home and sit up with pillows to support my back for the rest of the day to allow the spine to "glue itself in place" so she would not need to adjust it again. Then she said my spine had been so overworked that she wanted me to go to bed and stay flat on my back for a week except for three short walks a day, and for me to wear very loose clothing with no elastic around my waist.

The upper spinal inversion caused by the first chiropractor was an additional injury she had to correct, however she too did not discover the misalignment in my Atlas. The adjustment itself was very painless and gentle. I lay face down on her table and she placed pillows underneath my chest and hips. She asked me to breathe deeply while she very gently massaged my spine around the inversion. After a time she helped me up and sent me home. I was too tired from sleep deprivation to speak to her about my thoughts on what was causing the pain originally. I just told her it began with an exercising injury at home.

I followed her instructions and found myself experiencing such excruciating pain throughout my ribs, back and spine that I nearly lost my mind. When I called her she explained the muscles and tendons were being stretched into the new position and this can cause a lot of pain. She suggested I try a small glass of wine. I went to bed and tried not to cry because it hurt so much, and finally got to sleep. In my follow-up visits with her, she said my back was holding and recommended a series of arm circles, neck stretches and tiger stretches to do at home. She also recommended swimming with a specific series of strokes and lots of rest. The swimming was difficult, but it felt good to strengthen and stretch my back as well as be back in the water again after having been an avid swimmer prior to the injury.

The exercises at home, particularly the neck stretches, dramatically exacerbated my pain and afterward my entire body would tremble and shake for several hours, forcing me into bed. I called this my "meltdown" where my husband had to lift me in and out of bed and provide major assistance. Because I did realize my Atlas was misaligned and the worst thing you can do with a C-1 subluxation is to exercise, stretch or massage your neck, I suffered many meltdowns. When I told her about the pain she reassured me that it was to be expected and would eventually get better. It did not.

I quit seeing her ten months later in December of 1994 after thirteen visits. I also discontinued her exercise protocol. I further reduced my ADLs (activities of daily living), rested a lot more and began to get a little better. However, as soon as I tried to do something normal like wash the dishes, I would immediately get worse again. I decided to stop chiropractic treatment for a time and just manage my pain by laying my head down and resting on my back a lot during the day. By this time I could only work a few hours a day because it was getting harder and more painful to hold up my head.

During 1995, I spent a lot of time resting in bed between activities – working part time in my business in fifteen minute increments on a timer and a couple hours a week for a man who ran a healing center in exchange for alternative methods of managing pain. He was using the "Rife Machine" to disrupt pain signals, delivering a low-voltage programmed electrical wave through the body in a very safe way and "germanium patches" that contained small discs of germanium (a brittle gray crystalline chemical element used as semiconductors and alloys).

Studies had shown that germanium is able to relieve pain by connecting broken energy circuits in the muscle, disburse energy congestion, heal aggravated nerves and return strength to the muscles. His method seemed to be helping and did not involve anything invasive, so I used it for most of that year. During that year I attempted to go back to studying voice, singing in small concerts and returned to performing small roles in local theaters, all of which I previously had to stop doing after my exercise accident at home in November of 1993. I immediately got worse again from the exertion of singing as I stretched my ribs during deep breathing, standing upright and moving while I sang. I still believed the problem was coming from my neck and spine so I decided to find another chiropractor.

On January 19, 1996 I consulted with a third chiropractor who used yet another method. I brought with me the x-rays taken in December of 1993 by the first chiropractor and after looking at them with me he remarked that they showed a perfectly aligned spine and the first chiropractor was wrong. After palpating my spine, he diagnosed a "flat upper spine where the ribs were not moving, and possible scar tissue." Later on he told me I was likely suffering from "myofascial pain syndrome" (chronic pain in the connective tissues) after he did some extensive reading online. He said that there was no known cause and recommended a treatment plan including adjustments two to three times a week with the activator method he used – a small instrument that delivered a pulse directly to the subluxation causing bones to move, muscles and connective tissues to relax, relieving pain.

He said the activator would not hurt me and was the gentlest method available. He explained this method would tear any scar tissue away from the muscle and regular massage done in his office prior to each adjustment would break up this scar tissue and allow the body to absorb it. He also told me that I should be well in three to four months. He did not recommend I get an MRI or further x-rays because they would not provide any more information and would not show scar tissue. He also gave me some specific back stretching and strengthening exercises. The treatments seemed to help with the pain and spasms for short periods of time, however I could not do the exercises because they seemed to exacerbate the pain, just as they did before.

Beginning in February 1996, I performed the lead role in *HMS Pinafore* at a local theater. During the seven-weekend run I saw my chiropractor three times a week and sometimes on the weekends between performances to relieve chronic back spasms and pain. I also used a lot of ice packs, and continued to use germanium patches all over my back to get through it. After the run was over (twenty-two performances) my condition had declined further and I was unable to work more than an hour or so a day. After months of massage and activator treatments trying to keep going, my central nervous system became so hyper-sensitized it got to the point where there was no relief anymore from the treatments, just more pain and spasms, mostly on the right side of my neck and back.

When I tried to express my deep concern that the treatment was not going as he predicted, he continued to insist that the activator should not be causing me any pain and I must go on with the adjustments and the massage to re-educate the muscles if I were to get well. I disagreed, much to his dismay. It seemed to me that he was honestly invested in helping me, but his activator method seemed somewhat of a religion to him. He could not open his mind to the possibility that his activator may be hurting me. After the last treatment in November of 1996 caused me so much pain and shaking that I could hardly talk, he finally admitted that in my case maybe the pulse of the activator could be hurting me. I decided to quit his treatments and leave yet another chiropractor and his promise of a cure.

Meanwhile, and after *HMS Pinafore* had closed, the local opera company offered me the lead role in the operetta *The Merry Widow* opening in November of 1996. It was the dream I had been working so hard toward for so many years and I simply could not turn it down. I felt I would find a way to get through it and do well anyway in spite of the pain. During rehearsals leading up to opening night and throughout each of the seven performances, I had to resort to the strongest over-the-counter anti-inflammatory available, in addition to prescription codeine. I knew there was no understudy and heard the opera company was spending $54,000.00 that had been donated by the community on the production and I did not want to let them down or miss the experience. I also intuitively knew that this would be the last chance in my life to perform a dream lead role in my dream profession.

I remember times when my fellow actors had to push me up the stairs to get me onto the stage. Once I was there the adrenaline rush helped me perform. After each performance I used frozen wet towels on my burning back muscles and remember the towels steaming after only one or two minutes. I took heavy anti-histamines to get to sleep at night and used a strong pain spray and ice patches on my back at all times. I also had to stay in bed day and night between rehearsals and performances.

During the time between September and December 1996, I also sought the help of an acupuncturist who diagnosed me with "myo-fibrosis" of the upper back (abnormal thickening and/or scarring of muscle and connective tissue following injury, infection, lack of oxygen or surgery). He said I had too much deep massage and too much manipulation of the spine. When he inserted the needles, it was abnormally painful and he remarked that the nerve pathways were hyper-sensitive throughout my back.

He recommended weekly acupuncture treatments, rest and arm lifts. The pain seemed to improve for a few hours after his treatments, however, what I had come to call "the spot" in my mid-back on the right side because it was still so chronically tight and painful, began to flare-up with sharp, burning pain after each treatment. I felt that the acupuncture was activating the nerves too much and the treatment was not going to help me after all, so I stopped going in December of 1996.

I managed to get through *The Merry Widow* without collapsing out of sheer willpower. I remember on closing night sitting in my dressing room surrounded by beautiful flowers, looking down at my dressing table at all of the bottles of pills and crying while I realized that I had to stop singing. I was in a daze, so overwhelmed and in so much pain I felt like I was going to go insane. By the time the show was over I was flat out on my back, and could no longer move or get out of bed because of the horrific back, neck, and shoulder pain and spasms, severe fatigue and brain fog, peptic ulcer disease from too much ibuprofen, constant migraine headaches, dizziness and sleep deprivation.

My skin was so tender I could not be touched without experiencing pain and the muscles in my back had become so chronically tight that they were pulling three to four ribs out constantly. My neck was so tight I could not bend it or turn my head to the left. By now I could no longer take a deep breath or get away from the pain, no matter what I did. My life had come to a screeching halt and I was completely disabled. I did not know it at the time, but things were about to go from bad to worse – much, much worse.

I still believed that the problem was in my neck and spine and had begun with the head injury from the auto accident over three decades earlier and further compounded by the 1993 accidental injury at home, yet still no one so far had taken my analysis seriously, told me why I was in so much pain, or given me any definitive diagnosis. I felt I had no choice at this point but to enter into the cult of the systemized medical profession and throw myself on their mercy.

I was about to become a system patient, analyzed by doctors whose heads were immersed in the modern trends of today's medical profession, and treated with the standard available treatments that most likely used pharmaceuticals with recommended dosages based on results from studies done on the average patient with similar symptoms. Since I had not yet received a clear diagnosis, it seemed ambiguous to me as to which set of symptoms I should seek treatment for first. I decided to begin with the central nervous system because it seemed to be presenting the most serious symptoms, and seek the opinion of a local neurologist.

On December 12, 1996 I went to a local neurologist for a consultation and exam, and was very curious to hear what he had to say. I reserved forty-five minutes of his time so I could tell him my story, show him my diagrams of my theory of cause and discuss his findings with him. He listened hastily, palpated my back and tested my nervous system by tapping my knee with a small rubber-tipped hammer. When he tapped my right knee my foot shot up and kicked him hard. He was amazed at the acute knee-jerk reaction and remarked that it measured off the charts.

He then curiously told me that my neurology seemed otherwise normal and imagined the cause of my symptoms was growing mysterious scar tissue for some unknown reason throughout my back. All he could offer was a prescription for a drug that would inhibit the growth of the presumed scar tissue. I told him that I could not understand why I would be growing scar tissue throughout my back after already having had extensive treatment to break up theoretical scar tissue and had experienced no broken bones or surgery.

When I declined the drug and wanted to discuss other options, he said he was very busy and had to go, recommended an MRI, lots of rest and if I was not better in one month to go see the doctors at the Spine Care Center in Daly City, California. He gave me the name of the doctors who were responsible for the treatment of Joe Montana's back, and sent me on my way. He was young, impatient, condescending, overstressed and treated me like a mental case. I felt I had wasted my time. In checking into various types of alternative medicine, I found out about another chiropractor an hour's drive away who had a long-standing reputation of being very kind, took his time listening to his patients, was a minimalist in his treatment plans, and was very well informed.

On December 20, 1996 I went to see this chiropractor after giving my options a lot of thought. When I arrived at his office he saw me from his window. I was being helped out of the car and making my way toward his front door carrying my x-rays from the first chiropractor in one hand and holding onto my mother who brought me with the other. He greeted me at the door and helped me into a treatment room and onto a table that had supportive pillows. He told me that he had never before seen anyone in so much pain.

He placed my x-rays up on a lighted board on the wall next to me. I briefly told him my story, gave him my verbal analysis and a copy of my drawings and waited patiently while he looked very carefully at the film. He took a few minutes to think about what he was seeing and what I said before he spoke. He said he thought the reason I was unable to bend my neck forward was the muscles in my neck were in such spasm that they would not allow my vertebra to move.

After another pause, he pointed carefully at the area on the x-rays at the top of my spine. He said if you look closely you see that the alignment is not quite right at the point where my spine met my skull. He told me he thought my problem was coming from a subluxation at the top of my spine (the Atlas). He admitted only knowing one method that realigned the entire spine at the same time, involving wrapping a towel around the top of my neck and pulling sharply in an upward direction. He felt uneasy about trying this with me because although it could possibly help me, it could also make me worse and since I had already been made worse by a number of treatments, he did not want to be another source of pain for me.

His diagnosis was: C-1 subluxation, right front clavicle was out, the second rib left of second thoracic vertebrae was out, and the eleventh rib on the right side of the eleventh thoracic vertebrae was also out. He remarked that the discs between the second, third and fourth vertebrae were cloudy and that this was due to compression from chronic muscle tension in the neck and shoulders, indicating early degenerative disc disease. He also noted the TMJ on the right side of my jaw and used his fingers to assert pressure on the area to relieve pain and spasm.

He decided to give me a heat treatment on a softly padded table with a special lamp while supporting my head with an alignment pillow to relieve the pressure on the spinal cord and relax the muscles. He was very careful and spent a long time with me. He aligned the noted subluxations with a minimal pulse from the activator but stated that because my back had been activated to death for ten months by the previous chiropractor with no lasting results, this form of treatment was clearly not fixing the problem.

He suggested micro-current testing and soft tissue treatment by an osteopath in Salinas, California, which was also closer to Monterey where I lived. I saw this chiropractor one more time, and decided to continue on my search. Since I was unable to get an appointment with the osteopath he referred me to until February of 1997, I went ahead and made an appointment for the first available time with the doctor at the Spine Care Clinic in Daly City who had been recommended to me. This became a decision that I would later regret.

On January 2, 1997 I went for an initial consultation with the doctor in Daly City, California who was supposed to have successfully repaired Joe Montana's back – the former quarterback for the San Francisco 49'ers. My husband took me to a nearby hotel the night before my appointment. The ride up lying down in the backseat of the car with pillows all around me was so difficult I was nauseous from the pain by the time I arrived and could not walk on my own. I spent the night crying, intermittently dozing and throwing up.

By morning my nervous system had calmed down enough to get in the car and go to a restaurant for breakfast. My mind was still fuzzy from the amount of pain signals it was receiving and it was very hard for me to form sentences and talk. Over breakfast my husband and I labored to put together a long list of my symptoms to present to the doctor. When we got to his office I was put into a treatment room to wait for the doctor. I chose to sit in a corner chair propped up against the wall with pillows behind my back, head and neck for cushion and support. The exam table was too hard.

When the doctor came into the room he suggested I lie down on the treatment table, I told him it would hurt too much to lie on such a firm surface. I handed him the x-rays from the first chiropractor and my list of symptoms. He gave me a general movement test and pressed on some areas around my neck and shoulders. He said the x-rays did not reveal anything to him and wanted to order a new cervical x-ray, cervical MRI and do a test called a cervical discography because he suspected I had two herniated discs in my neck and he needed these tests to confirm his suspicion. Then, another doctor, apparently the one that was chief in the care of Joe Montana came in for a very brief consultation, leaving shortly after concurring with the first doctor's suspicions.

I asked the doctor who was apparently in charge to review the list of my symptoms I had so painstakingly put together and his reply was, "I am not going to discuss seventy-five scenarios from a list of possible symptoms until I get the results of these tests!" I felt shot down and shut out, but I was too weak and too foggy to argue with him. He then gave me a foam neck brace, a prescription for 500mg of Vicodin painkiller to take four times a day, 20mg of Valium muscle-relaxer to take twice a day and a sleep aid to take at night. He did not warn me that Vicodin and Valium were highly addictive. I made an appointment for February 7, 1997 for the x-rays, MRI and the discography to be done at Seaton Medical Center below the Spine Care Clinic, filled my prescriptions at their in-house pharmacy and went home.

During the interim between appointments, I took the prescriptions as ordered and fell into a deep fog of mental haze and dulled pain. I wore the neck brace each time I got up from bed and felt nauseated after taking the Vicodin painkiller, but the Valium muscle-relaxer kept me from throwing up. I was still in a kind of miserable pain and was also becoming severely constipated from the drug regimen. My stool was becoming hard like rocks and was very painful. It caused tearing and bleeding in my rectum. Little did I know that I was also becoming addicted to Vicodin and Valium. The peptic ulcer disease was not improving either and was getting so bad that I began throwing up the bland food I was trying to eat.

I had to put myself on a baby food diet and supplemented with warm milk toast. I could not brush my own teeth or hair or shave my legs anymore. I could hardly do anything for myself at all, and it became especially hard because my husband still had to go to work every day. I was alone for some very long hours. One or two people helped me from time-to-time, but that was the exception. I really had to manage by myself for the most part and spent the majority of my days lying back on the recliner propped heavily with pillows watching old movies and dozing off in a foggy haze of pain, trying not to throw up.

On February 7, 1997 my husband took me back up to Daly City to see the doctor at the Spine Care Clinic and have the cervical MRI and discography done. After checking in at the clinic I was sent downstairs where the tests would be performed. First I underwent the MRI and the results were sent to the doctor. We went back upstairs to see the doctor briefly and he said the MRI showed that the discs were cloudy which indicated compression and early degenerative disc disease but that they were not herniated as he originally suspected.

He then said he still wanted to see the results of the discography before he made his final determination. Although there was no indication on the MRI of a ruptured or bulging disc, he explained he still wanted the discography to tell him whether or not he was right about his original suspicion that the problem was coming from this area. We went back downstairs where I was admitted and taken to a dressing room just beyond the nurse's station. I was given a robe to put on while my husband waited in the waiting room. I was asked to lie on a padded table and prepared with 20mg of intravenous Valium, an antibiotic and a saline drip.

After a time I was wheeled into a procedure room and the technician who was going to do the discography came up to me and introduced himself. He told me I would be given a hypnotic drug just before the procedure to help me forget the experience. I asked him to explain how the procedure was done. He said the vocal chords would be pushed to one side and a fluid would be injected into each disc between C-1 and C-5 through a four-inch needle inserted from the front of my neck. The pressure of the fluid into the discs was supposed to temporarily worsen my symptoms of pain and in theory would show the problem was coming from the discs. That was when the fight or flight alarms really began to sound inside me, and terror was written all over my face.

I fought through the Valium with the help of an extreme adrenaline rush and asked the technician to look at my MRI and tell me what percentage he thought likely that the problem was coming from my discs. After careful consideration and looking at my MRI and x-rays, he was kind enough to honestly say in his opinion the chances of the problem coming from my discs were roughly ten percent or less. I then asked him if he read in my chart and saw I was an opera singer and if there was any chance this procedure could do permanent damage to my vocal chords. He said yes, there was about a twenty percent chance that this could happen.

I suddenly felt intensely nauseated and I began to hyperventilate. The technician saw in spite of the Valium, I was beginning to have a panic attack and he took my hand and said, "You know, you do not have to do this if you don't want to."

I was hardly able to talk and had begun crying, but I made myself say to him, "The doctor said he would not discuss my symptoms until after he had the results of the discography."

The technician then became noticeably angry and said, "You just lie here quietly while I go upstairs and have a talk with the doctor."

After he left I waited a few minutes, feeling sick and afraid. A nurse came in and asked me how I was doing and I said that I was not going to have the procedure after all, and asked her if she would please wheel me out into the holding area in front of the nurse's station while I waited for the technician to return. She did, and while I was lying there waiting I saw a middle-aged Caucasian man sitting in a wheelchair all slumped over with a dark, sunken, pain-ridden face trying to charm the nurses into giving him more painkillers. I knew then this was hell on earth and decided it was not going to be where I would end up. In one motion I pulled the IV out of my arm, rolled off the table onto the floor and crawled down the hallway to the dressing room. I slowly got dressed on the floor and crawled up the wall, using it to support me as I made my way to the waiting room to find my husband. It amazes me to this day that not one person at that busy nurse's station saw me do this.

When I located my husband I said to him, "Get me out of here, I can't do this." He put his arms around me and helped me to the elevator and out to the car. I lay down in the backseat with my pillows and we left for home. It was nightfall by then, and that night there was a rainstorm to end all rainstorms and the valleys between Daly City and Monterey around Watsonville were all flooding. The highway had a detour that provided an alternate route along the hills and the traffic was heavy and slow. The car was going through two inches of water and it took four hours to make what should have been a one and a half hour trip. When we got home I fell into bed and stayed there.

I felt I had just saved my own life, that in my weakened state combined with the hyper-sensitized state of my central nervous system, I knew I would not have survived the doctor's horrific experiment. I felt that I was badly treated by him, that his ego was too large to open his mind to my insights, and that he had become jaded by experiencing so many people in pain. I also felt his expertise as a surgeon had narrowed his vision so his options had become severely limited.

He was a product of a system of "diagnosing by exclusion" so commonly used in diagnosing chronic FMS without offering himself the benefit of updating his knowledge on his own. He seemed to know nothing about FMS. He had no clue what was really wrong with me and should have admitted this before risking my well-being to satisfy his curiosity. He should have referred me to someone who might know more than he did about chronic pain syndromes.

On February 11, 1997 I had my initial consultation with the osteopath that was referred to me by the kind chiropractor in Hollister, California. By this time my condition had deteriorated to a point where I was so weak I could only speak in a whisper and I was beginning to believe I was dying. I had to be helped into the office from a prone position in the car. I was put in the waiting room for a time and then I had to be helped to slowly walk from the waiting room into the treatment room. I remember having to stop every few steps because my entire body would spasm and tighten up like a giant convulsion, and then after breathing through it, the spasms would release for another few steps and then it would happen again. The people in the waiting room were all looking at me with grave concern.

My entire body was in so much pain and spasm, bending was nearly impossible. The doctor and a nurse helped me up onto a treatment table and he spent an hour with me taking my history and examining me. He ordered a number of blood tests and told me he wanted to admit me into the hospital immediately. I became very agitated at the thought and my heart rate and breathing began to escalate into a panic attack. I said as clearly as I could with my weak voice that I did not want to go into the hospital and be at the mercy of a group of doctors and nurses who have not been able to diagnose me after all that had happened, let alone listen to me. I meant no disrespect, but by now I was very weary and afraid of being mistreated again by the medical professionals that I believed almost killed me. He said he understood completely and told me that I had been a victim of medical abuse and was extremely over medicated and exacerbated, I was in an extreme dissociative state.

The osteopath recommended reducing my meds beginning immediately and told me that he wanted me to see a homeopath in Watsonville as soon as I was able to. He wanted to begin a schedule of osteopathic manipulations to the muscle tissue beginning in five days and have me come in twice a week for a couple weeks, then once a week, then once every two weeks for a while. He felt he could relieve the muscle tension and increase circulation into what he described as sludgy and toxic muscle tissue throughout my back, shoulders and neck.

He seemed genuinely concerned, however when he said he thought he could get me where he wanted me to be in about ten treatments, I instinctively knew he probably had no experience with someone in my condition. It was quite obvious to me that it would take a lot more than ten osteopathic manipulations to get me well. He also wanted to start me on a single neurotransmitter reuptake inhibitor called Nortriptaline that deals with balancing the brain chemical norapinephrine involved in chronic pain, but did not prescribe it yet. He gave me an order for lab tests to be done close to home.

On February 16, 1997 I went to see the osteopath again. However during the five-day interim between appointments with him, I became so distressed about having been overly medicated I decided to throw all my pills down the toilet, not having any idea I had been taking a high dosage of a very addictive narcotic in Vicodin for about six weeks. Within a couple of days, I began to suffer from severe withdrawals and I felt like my body was slowly being drawn through a white-hot paper shredder. My entire body was convulsing non-stop and I was in so much pain I could barely talk.

The heaviest point of the withdrawals came during the second night after I stopped taking Vicodin. My husband held me in his arms for several hours. When the morning came, it was the day I was supposed to go and see the doctor for the second time. When I arrived at his office, my mother went in and got help to get me into the office through the back-door and straight into a treatment room. The nurse's aid on duty came in and saw me trembling and in severe pain and asked me if I was going through heroin withdrawals. I said, "What! What are you talking about? All I did was stop taking my pain medication."

The doctor came in soon after and took one look at me and said, "You are worse! What has happened?" I told him that I had thrown all my medication into the toilet and he gasped and said, "You cannot stop taking an addictive narcotic cold-turkey! You are going through severe withdrawals and this is very dangerous!" I said, "What do you mean? No one told me that Vicodin was an addictive narcotic. No one!" I told him I did not want to go back on the Vicodin and he told me he would prescribe a milder narcotic that would help me get off it safely.

He examined me again and found my back was on fire. I was in a cold, clammy sweat, my heart rate was way up and my breathing was labored. He gave me a prescription for Darvocet, and since I had not made it to the lab between visits, he gave me another order for the blood tests to be done that afternoon. He wanted to see me again in a few days after the results were back and then he would begin the osteopathic manipulation therapy (OMT) on my musculature.

My mother and I left and went straight to the lab. Three lab technicians helped me from the car into the lab and to put me on a table to draw some blood. Two of them had to hold me steady because I was shaking so severely while the other one drew the blood. Then we went to the pharmacy where I waited in the car for the medication and as soon as it was filled I took a pill with some water on the spot. It only took about twenty minutes before things eased up and I stopped shaking. When I got home I went to bed and stayed there for what seemed to be days and days, taking the Darvocet on schedule every four hours and waiting for that third hour when the withdrawal symptoms would return until twenty minutes after I took the next pill.

I had to endure one hour and twenty minutes of horrible withdrawals near the end of every four-hour interval round the clock for three weeks. After two weeks the withdrawal time at the third hour's end seemed to get easier and I was finally able to get some sleep. When I got stronger I would see the doctor again and begin the OMT of the toxic muscle tissue in my back, neck and shoulders. But for the time being I was "strung out," exhausted and very, very weak, but was still fiercely determined to get off all the medication given to me by the doctor at Spine Care Clinic. All I was taking at this point was the Darvocet.

On February 30, 1997 I got back to the osteopath to begin the OMT and it was also time to start the Nortriptaline. He told me about the results of the blood test and said that I did not have Lupus or Rheumatoid Arthritis, and I did not have an infection. He said the rest of the results were unremarkable. I talked further about my history focusing on the car accident that I had three decades ago. I gave him a copy of the related diagram I had drawn in 1993 of what I considered to be the cause of what seemed like a central nervous system neurological malfunction. He took the diagram, looked at it briefly and filed it away in the back of my file for the time being, and I thought he would get back to it later on.

His first OMT treatment was really remarkable. He concentrated on my neck and released a spasm on the left side that had prevented me from turning my head to the left for over a year. I remembered the chiropractor in Hollister told me he thought this osteopath was very talented. Then the osteopath gently pulled on my ankles and lifted my legs to stretch my spine and my legs lit up like buzzing power lines. Osteopaths are trained in energy and tactile sensitivity and are also said to be able to feel a pea under a pile of phone books. He remarked about how much excess energy there was in my legs. He wanted to work on another area the next time and I made a series of appointments according to his protocol.

I left his office feeling like his treatments might help my muscle health and eventually increase my mobility, but I was cautious about whether or not he could help the pain. He gave me a prescription for the Nortriptaline and told me it will take my body about three weeks to adjust to it before the benefits showed up. He also told me that the adjustment period might be a bit challenging. I filled the prescription on the way home and began taking it immediately.

I did go through a couple weeks or so of some nausea, dizziness and increased nightmares on top of the regular symptoms, but I eventually got used to the drug and these side effects gradually went away. I chose to ignore this doctor's comment about the idea that I was imagining my side affects after his suggestion that I not read the bottle listing them. The drug seemed to help the depression a bit but I felt no measurable relief from the pain and spasms. I called the homeopath he had recommended to me and made an appointment to see him. The homeopath was located forty-five minutes away so someone had to take me. He was a classical constitutional homeopath and an osteopath as well, and had abandoned the medical profession because of their gross overuse of drugs and their extreme limitations. He now devoted all of his time to homeopathic medicine and no longer practiced osteopathy.

On March 13, 1997 I saw the homeopath for the first time. He spent about two hours total with me taking my history and talking with me about my condition, my life and my relationships. After the initial interview he took me into an examining room, helped me onto a treatment table and palpated my back muscles. He said he understood what I had and the solution was homeopathy and osteopathy. He called my condition "Neuromuscular facilitation with resting potential set too high." In other words I had chronically tight muscles that never relaxed.

Later on when I asked him if I had FMS, he said he believed I did not and that my condition was more like Myofascial Pain Syndrome. Since then I have discovered Myofascial Pain Syndrome is one of the symptoms of FMS. He concluded his analysis by matching me to a constitutional remedy and on April 15, 1997, I began my homeopathic treatment with a single 200c dose with a 6c dose to take daily to keep it going strong. The remedy seemed to help for a short while, for about two weeks, by lessoning the pain about 25%, but I was not getting better overall.

On June 5, 1997 he changed my remedy with a 200c dose of another and a 6c daily because I was not improving enough, and I took this for a little over six months. I remember having some very heavy emotional releases and horrific nightmares that were very dark, graphic and bloody. I was having such a difficult time psychologically he recommended a psychologist to "bridge the gap" between what was being released and what I was able to understand. He knew of a psychologist in my area who specialized in victims of psychological trauma and referred me to her. I was still unable to walk more than a few feet by myself, but I agreed to go and see her.

It was simply a matter of getting myself to my car, driving there and sitting up with pillows for fifty minutes. This was no easy task but I knew it would help me move forward. I had been to a psychologist before who told me that my mother was a young girl and that my father did not uphold his 50% responsibility in raising me. She also told me I needed to set some boundaries in my dysfunctional relationships. I decided I wanted more information and was interested in learning all I could about psychological health.

On July 24, 1997 I had my first appointment with the new psychologist. Since I could not afford to see her more than once a month I came prepared with a list of events outlining my life in general and the people involved. After reading it and talking with me, she explained my family's dysfunction and that they were made that way through childhood circumstances beyond their control through no fault of their own. She recommended I read a book entitled *"Trapped In The Mirror"* by Elan

Golomb, Ph.D. She also recommended that I read *"Toxic Parents"* by Dr. Susan Forward in the time between appointments.

Before I left she got down on the floor where I was lying and drew a diagram of the protective wall children of dysfunctional parents often build. She outlined on paper the adapted child inside the wall. This was all new to me and she wanted me to keep coming, so I agreed. She said my most important and most immediate goal for getting well was to emotionally detach from the dysfunctional relationships in my life as completely and as soon as possible, and not to ever attempt to communicate with them about the past. She warned me that my sibling could not be trusted to be safe or respectful, and was very likely to have a violent psychological reaction to my actions.

She suggested I not speak to any family member about my therapy or who my therapist was, or explain to anyone why I was detaching because no one in my family was likely to respect my decision, behave appropriately by minding their own business, or be safe psychologically. I clearly understood that boundaries of space and time would be indicating a move in my position and that I was going to be perceived as a threat. Dysfunctional people believe they can behave as they wish toward others without consequences or without ever taking personal responsibility. This was a moral standard I no longer wanted to be a part of. I needed to become healthy psychologically and I wanted my health to be rooted in reality, not destructive fantasies. I finally found the path to becoming a healthy, happy adult and was anxious to take responsibility for my own life and do whatever was necessary to get well.

So I bought the books and began reading them. I could not sit up in a chair nor could I hold up a book so I read them lying on my back in bed, putting the books on a pillow on my chest. I rested my arms to each side of the open book, propping it up between my limp hands and pillow. I was only able to read a few pages at a time but I was so determined to get the first book read by the time I had my next session. The process began with my learning to understand the degrees in which my parents were psychologically compromised and how common varying degrees of dysfunction exist in most families in our society.

I also learned how unhealthy it was to maintain a position in dysfunctional relationships without boundaries or a clear sense of self. My therapist was very reassuring that I could learn all I needed to in order to be healthy as long as I had the willingness. During the course of my two years in therapy I read over forty books on human psychology and health supervised by my therapist. I also underwent two sessions in EMDR (Eye Movement Desensitization and Reprocessing) that were both extremely successful in neutralizing my symptoms from Post-Traumatic Stress Disorder caused by childhood and early life experiences.

At the time my psychological education began, my homeopath began to take me on what turned out to be a four-year wild goose chase for the right remedy. Between April 17, 1997 and June 17, 2001 this homeopath had given me nineteen separate hits of 200c doses with 6c daily doses, and eleven separate hits of an LM-1 dose, for a total of eleven different remedies. These remedies at these doses were not doing what he wanted them to and at times were making me worse.

On June 17, 2001 he reverted back to my original remedy and this would turn out to be my last visit with this homeopath. They say that a good homeopath should be able to match you to the right remedy at the dose in the first few tries, many times on the first visit. I was clearly frustrated and so was he. My pain was better overall in some ways but I was still unable to do anything. After four years of this homeopath honestly trying to help me, I was still housebound from pain and too disabled to work or keep house.

I had been in counseling from July of 1997 until July of 1999 and I had learned a great deal. During this time I separated myself from those I needed to for self-preservation and had set boundaries with others who needed them. My homeopath had still been unable to find the right remedy for me and his final conclusion was, "I feel that your hyper-vigilance in your record keeping and in your personality has prevented the remedies I have tried from working."

The truth is I had naturally become hyper-vigilant because we had been going around in circles for four years and because I was still very ill and felt my chances of getting well depended on how accurately I was able to record my symptoms and my reactions to each remedy. It had become apparent that because his treatment plan had failed, he chose to blame his failure elsewhere.

On October 10, 2001 I wrote him a letter and told him that I felt it was time for me to have my case reviewed by another homeopath after more than four years of searching for the correct remedy with him and not finding it.

On October 30, 2001 I saw my current homeopath for the first time. She was very impressed after reading the long list of remedies and the dosages used on me that I was still willing to have an open mind towards the field.

I told her just because I had not seen the right homeopath did not mean the principle of homeopathy was unsound. I was still going to an osteopath for OMT on my muscles, but had changed osteopaths in February of 2001 to a local DO closer to home. The OMT treatments had been helping manage my muscle pain and tension, had increased mobility and brought more circulation into the soft tissues so they became healthier, but it had not done very much to relieve the CNS pain and had not been curative. It was time to change homeopaths and osteopaths.

I told my new homeopath that my first osteopath was so uninformed about FMS that he once told me I should go for a walk in the mall to get my mind off my problems at a time when I was too sick and in too much pain to walk around the house. I was glad to change to my current osteopath who is a kind and understanding man who has always been willing to listen to me and work with me. Although he did not initially believe homeopathy had been helping me, it still made sense to believe in combining homeopathy with osteopathy.

After a two-hour interview with my new homeopath, she told me I did not appear on the outside to be as compromised as I actually was, but she could see that underneath the innate vitality and strength I projected on the surface, I was very, very ill. She said she could see how a doctor could be fooled by my appearance because I did not appear to be anywhere near as sick as I was.

Four years later she shared her initial impression of me when we first met as she said to herself, "Now there's a powerhouse!" At our first visit she explained that although she could see I was a highly sensitive individual, she could also see that I was an incredibly strong person, and that sensitivity and strength were different things.

She also said my instincts were very good and I should never hesitate to follow them. Then she said my former homeopath never understood exactly how sensitive and compromised I was because he was probably fooled by my outward appearance. She said he should never have given me a 200c dose of any remedy or a 6c daily dose, nor should I have ever been given any LM dose.

She explained these doses were way too high for someone with my sensitivity who was as compromised as I was, and I should have been given no more than a single 12c dose to begin with. She also said he hit on the right remedy a couple of times but because his doses were too high, all they did was aggravate my condition and mask any possible benefit that could have been derived from the remedy.

She explained further that a highly sensitive and weakened organism absolutely could not be bombarded with a 200c dose of remedy and never given an LM. She went on to say that Dr. Hahnemann, the German father of homeopathy, said over 200 years ago with regard to dosage, "The least amount should be given to the organism to initiate forward movement and build strength slowly. Too much will only serve to exacerbate the symptoms and block healing."

It became very clear to me that this was what I had been going through, but I had been so dependant on this treatment psychologically for lack of any other visible alternatives and had felt some degree of relief, I was too desperate and afraid to question it. I even think now I was in a kind of denial out of the fear that I might never get well.

My new homeopath said she knew of the man who had been treating me and that all of the patients that came to her after being with him were afraid. She said she was not so strict and did not believe in giving everyone a 200c dose. She gave me some literature on antidoting precautions and then told me my remedy was Belladonna. On October 30, 2001 she began by giving me a 12c dose with no daily dose, told me to go home, get a lot of rest and allow time for the remedy to begin working. I felt so reassured and very relieved because she had made so much sense in breaking down my previous experience. For the first time I began to relax and believe I was truly on the right path. I just needed to find the right doctor to help me along my way.

On January 24, 2002 my homeopath felt I was strong enough to be given a 30c dose and continued giving me one 30c dose every few months through June 11, 2004. In March of 2002 I had improved enough for my osteopath to refer me to a warm water physical therapy pool in town to go twice a week. I was growing stronger and beginning to feel better overall. On June 21, 2002 I had Lasik surgery on my eyes. In March of 2003 I was able to undergo a colonoscopy. In November of 2003 my husband and I took a two-day get-a-way trip by car and another in February of 2004 to our favorite coastal town near Hearst Castle. I was still crashing a lot energetically and flaring up when I would overdo it, but I was beginning to recover a little faster each time and was starting to get a little more out of life.

From June of 2004 through the end of 2005 my homeopath gave me a couple different remedies to heal the layers that were presenting themselves. By January of 2006 I had become strong enough to be given a 200c dose of Belladonna, another 200c dose in September of 2006, and another in June of 2007. In November of 2007 I broke out with a small presentation of Shingles (Herpes Zoster) on the right side of my abdomen so she gave a 200c dose of Murcurius Vivus to heal it. The outbreak healed up in three weeks, remained minimal and in April of 2008 she put me back on a 200c dose of Belladonna after I had seven amalgam fillings in my mouth replaced with plastic. The homeopathy was working.

I had continued with the osteopathic treatments until November of 2002 at which time I decided to stop the OMT because I felt I no longer needed it. When I first saw my new osteopath in February of 2001, I was so ill I had agreed to a temporary protocol of drug therapy consisting of a painkiller, a muscle relaxer, an anti-inflammatory and the anti-depressant Prozak to break the pain and spasm cycle I was in at that time. I took the first three drugs until February of 2002 and then tapered off of them very quickly.

After more research I decided to change the antidepressant I had been taking for pain and depression from Prozak – a single neurotransmitter reuptake inhibiter like Nortriptaline, to a "dual neurotransmitter reuptake inhibitor" I had learned about called Cymbalta. Prozak had only worked with the neurotransmitter serotonin, as Nortriptaline had only worked with the neurotransmitter norepinephrine, the two principle neurotransmitters of sympathetic nerve endings to the major organs and skin.

Cymbalta is called a dual-inhibitor because it works with both of these principle neurotransmitters that are involved in pain and depression. Studies have shown that Cymbalta is more effective for many chronic pain patients in reducing pain signals in a hyper-sensitized central nervous system than single neurotransmitter drugs. However I was not ready to begin taking Cymbalta until November of 2005 and in time it proved to work better than the Nortriptaline or the Prozak I had tried earlier.

During a time when I was applying for Social Security Disability Benefits – which were denied because SS does not recognize FMS – my osteopath had made a remark in a letter to them about what he had palpated to be a severely misaligned Atlas vertebra. This jumped out at me because it fit with my assertion that the root cause of my condition was due to a blow on the head in an auto accident decades prior compounded by a neck injury at home nine years ago, resulting in a severe enough degree of Atlas misalignment to trigger full blown chronic FMS. So I asked him if he could recommend a chiropractor who could do a corrective Atlas adjustment. He gave me the name of someone he knew locally. In September of 2002 I saw this chiropractor for the first time. I was very excited to see this new chiropractor and on our first visit he listened to my theory of cause with great interest and completely agreed with it. He began what he called a conservative Atlas alignment treatment plan consisting of adjusting the Atlas once a week and would begin to taper off when it began to lock down. It turned out that an adjustment was needed once a week for five months before we could begin tapering off. This was helping me become more functional and was raising my ADLs (activities of daily living) slowly as time went on, but I was still leveling off at too low a level of functionality. This told me something important.

My symptoms would always begin to improve right after my adjustment, but because my Atlas would begin to slowly slip back out toward the old deviant position within a few days after each adjustment, my symptoms would begin to return again. Although I knew I was on the right track I did not seem to be getting beyond a certain point and was not improving enough to become more functional as time went by. My chiropractor took my 1995 diagram and my analysis very seriously and he understood the importance of aligning my Atlas, so we kept on trying.

In June of 2005 I learned from a friend about a chiropractor in South Lake Tahoe who had opened a Fibromyalgia Relief Clinic who was doing daily Atlas alignments on patients with chronic FMS and getting incredible results. His protocol of two to three adjustments per day for a time was very aggressive. I did not feel I wanted to do it quite that much, but I knew I needed more adjustments than I was getting. I talked about it with my chiropractor and we decided to abandon the conservative treatment plan and go for a slightly more aggressive one. I decided I wanted to try one adjustment a day until my Atlas held and then taper down slowly from there. I said, "Let's go for it!" and he said, "OK! Let's go!"

I did not expect my chiropractor to look into his crystal ball and give me a time line because I knew my body would heal in its own time. It did not matter anyway. I knew this was the right thing to do and all I wanted was to begin. I knew after my Atlas began to hold for longer periods of time my central nervous system would begin to do some real healing and this would take whatever time it would take. I also knew there would be ups and downs each time I increased my level of ADLs through this alignment process as my body gained strength and stamina, this was to be expected.

So in June of 2005 I began daily adjustments to align my Atlas. Soon after I began I had to quit my warm water pool exercise after going twice a week for over three years. The warm water was wonderful and had done me so much good but it was time to graduate. The next step was to exercise on land up against gravity. I chose a gentle Thai Chi class once a week and practiced at home between classes. I felt this was a good place to start. My daily adjustments went for three months and gradually my Atlas began to lock down. The thin muscles and tiny ligaments holding the Atlas in place had been stretched out for thirteen years and because they have memory, they wanted to move it back out into the old deviant position after each adjustment and were not yet strong enough to hold it in.

Prior to beginning the more aggressive Atlas alignment protocol, I had not been able to hold my head up for more than a couple hours, or even be up out of bed for more than a few hours at a time due to the stubborn way the Atlas would slip back out again after each adjustment. I was starting to stay out of bed for longer periods of time while the muscles learned to adhere to alignment and be re-educated by the protocol. In addition to the daily adjustments, I also received some gentle periodic massages prior to treatment to re-educate the muscles in my back that had been chronically constricted to relax and get used to the new positions of my neck, head and spine.

Life was beginning to change for the better in a very gradual manner as my central nervous system began healing and my body began gaining strength and stamina. To help the process along, my homeopath – who is also a chiropractor – suggested I allow her to do two separate twenty minute ultra-sound treatments on my back, followed by a back massage, acupressure work on my neck and ending with an Atlas adjustment. I scheduled two of these treatments three weeks apart in May and June of 2005, and I found that they helped a great deal.

After three months of daily adjustments, the C-1 vertebra was beginning to hold most of the time. By September of 2005 we began tapering off and by November of 2005 we went to every ten or eleven days for the next four months. November of 2005 was when I began taking Cymbalta prescribed by my osteopath to replace the Prozak he had me on earlier.

In March of 2006 my chiropractor began tapering off further and by April of 2006 we went to once every two weeks. During this time I experienced varied degrees of slippage in my Atlas (between 1mm and 4mm) depending on how well I remembered to keep my head in a neutral position and only turn it left to right no more than forty-five degrees, and how much new activity I added to my ADLs. I continued to increase normal activities while keeping up with weekly Thai Chi.

It was so interesting to observe each time I reached a new level of ADLs, my Atlas would slip a bit more frequently, but gradually the muscles accepted the new demands to hold it in place. Because the alignment must be exact, even slipping out one or two millimeters can cause a degree of symptoms to return. Understanding this in advance as the logical and natural course back to a healthy neck and spine prevented me from becoming discouraged when I experienced it. I learned early on that no one heals in an upward straight line. It always begins with ups and downs, two steps forward and one step back and increased from there in the same fashion.

My central nervous system had clearly begun to show signs of healing at this point. I was sleeping better all the time in a restful and restorative manner, my mind was clearing up, my energy level was continuing to increase and I was feeling better overall. These improvements included a gradual decrease in restless leg syndrome, decrease in overall buzzing, an increase in normal bowel function, a more normal acid balance in my stomach –thus better digestion, a marked decrease in migraine headaches, less and less nerve pain, muscle pain, soft tissue tightness and spasms and the psychological relief of seeing an end to this nightmare.

My long state of depression had lifted by this time and thoughts of suicide to escape the pain were now a distant memory. The pain flare-ups that were such a regular part of life finally began to disappear.

From August of 2006 through December of 2006, my chiropractor tapered off the adjustments to once a month for while to see how I did. Keeping the Atlas aligned within two to three millimeters, we were now able to settle on an efficient interval that kept it from slipping too far out between visits. At the same time I continued to gradually increase my ADLs. The interval we settled on became three weeks between adjustments and was a tricky balance to maintain as I became more and more active. By now I was no longer having painful flare-ups, my restless leg syndrome and overall buzzing was gone, the chronic spasms in the right side of my back had relaxed, the migraine headaches were gone and my tender points were nearly gone as well.

By January of 2006 my Atlas was holding in place with no more than one to two millimeters of slippage between visits and I was feeling like moving up a level in my ADLs in the near future. My chiropractor warned me to never use weights or lift anything heavy because doing so could strain the neck, shoulders and upper back, which would pull on the Atlas. By March of 2007 I had quit Thai Chi and began a class in gentle restorative yoga once a week at our local sports center. I kept up the once every three-week adjustment protocol with my chiropractor while my body adapted to the new demands of the yoga class.

By April of 2007 I felt strong enough to add one more restorative yoga class per week and ended up with a routine of yoga on Wednesdays and Fridays and a visit to my chiropractor every three weeks on a Monday. This routine became a winning formula. Yoga began rehabilitating my body toward overall balance and increased circulation to allow more oxygen and nutrients to reach soft tissues. It created healthier muscles that were lengthened and strengthened with increased flexibility and mobility. Yoga also enabled me to keep moving forward toward taking back my life without any more major setbacks.

Throughout this process there was some natural, temporary increases in pain. When I began Thai Chi my legs and back hurt more the first few weeks because the practice is done on your feet and relies on leg and upper back strength, but this eventually decreased to a normal amount of soreness the day after each practice. When I began yoga my upper back felt the brunt of the pain because the practice stretched connective tissues between my ribs and shoulder blades that had been chronically tight for many years and had developed a pattern of maintaining this tension and were also atrophied.

Gradually the connective tissues began to respond to the painful re-peated stretching during each yoga practice and eventually the pain turned into normal soreness for a day or so after class. I understood there was going to be some pain with the gain and I did not fret about it. I simply decided to go with the flow and accept that this stage too would pass as each stage had passed throughout the journey to healing this con-dition. Now, the light at the end of the tunnel clearly lit the way to my un -relinquished goal and this kept me from bowing my head or becoming weary.

I continued on with my treatment schedule, adding to my ADLs as often as I could, writing more in this book, etc., until one day in July of 2008 I received a call from another local chiropractor's office offering a promotion of a free consultation and x-rays with their doctor who was an upper cervical spine specialist. He had all the up-to-date equipment for doing the special Atlas subluxation x-ray, a special side "posture head drop table" for adjusting the Atlas, and nerve impulse measurement tech-nology that included a colored graph of your spine showing where the pain signals were coming from and their intensity.

I had been feeling stuck at the level I was on with my current chiro-practor for a while, and felt another change was needed, and voila, the universe sent me the perfect opportunity to get a fresh opinion. I made an appointment with the new doctor immediately, got evaluated and x-rayed and discovered something that was vital to my getting all the way well.

Of course, he identified my Atlas as having been a serious problem and showed me that my neck was angled to the left on the x-ray, along with a right head tilt that was not too drastic, but visible. He even showed me an actual human Atlas vertebra and how it was formed. This was amazing to me. He reviewed my case with me and when he listened to my story, the description of my theory of cause of FMS and how I had been treated thus far, he said I sounded like a chiropractor myself. He was astonished at what I knew and when I remarked that the Atlas was everything, he smiled and shook his head yes and said, "Yes, it is every-thing!"

He said my Atlas was locked in a forward subluxation and doubted the manual techniques my previous chiropractor had been using would dislodge the forward subluxation to completely realign the C-1 with the C -2 below. However he did say that his method had probably been suc-cessful in correcting the left shift of the Atlas, but it would not stay at 100% alignment between adjustments because the forward shift had not been unlocked. This made perfect sense to me. He showed me his "Atlas alignment side posture head drop table" and said it was developed specifically for adjusting this very subluxation.

He had me lie on the table on my side, bend my bottom arm at the elbow and lay my hand over my chest and my upper arm along my side and hip. He placed the side of my head in a groove on the head-rest, raised the separated portion of the table under my head with a foot peddle and then snapped that part of the table back down. I felt a jolt and an energy surge through my body, but it was not painful. It was just loud, and I felt a bit headachy afterward. Not a big deal at all, but it felt like something very profound had just happened.

I was really thrilled. He had me turn over and did the same on the other side. He helped me up and I walked slowly with my head level and straight to a quite room where I went to bed with nice neck pillow to support my head for about twenty minutes. I felt very good about what had just happened and I was optimistic about the results. It all made so much sense and provided a sound reason why I had leveled off short of being cured with my former chiropractor. He sent me home with some simple and sensible instructions and I was anticipating great results.

I continued going to him every three weeks for another year as I increased my ADLs, he explained that he needed to check my Atlas and lower neck and back as it adapted itself to the Atlas becoming stabilized at the top of my spine. Amazingly, in the first seven months of his treatment I only needed my Atlas adjusted five times, which seemed like a miracle to me. I was improving at a new rate and rapidly increasing activities, working more on this book, continuing yoga class twice a week, adding daily yoga at home, and adding a daily one-mile power walk. Much to my extreme pleasure and amazement, after six months of his treatment I was able to return to the water and began swimming laps again!

I'll never forget the first time I returned to the water after having been unable to swim without pain since my compounding neck injury 16 years earlier that had triggered full-blown chronic FMS. Prior to this critical accident I had been an avid swimmer, tennis player, bike rider and singer, but FMS very quickly forced me to stop all forms of exertion. I will never forget floating on my back while doing the backstroke that first time. I stopped and stared up at the sports center ceiling, I felt the velvety water all around me like a sacred womb and began to sob with happiness and gratitude. It was a major turning point in my recovery and I knew for certain I was coming back to myself. I knew that I would make it all the way. I was approaching the end of a long, dark tunnel after following what had begun as a faint light that was now becoming more miraculous, wonderful and more brilliant as it grew closer.

I still go to my chiropractor for a "tune-up" once in a while because I like to work hard at being strong and healthy and continue to cross-train with my three favorite exercises; yoga, power-walking and swimming. Through all the years of this process, I kept up my vigil of a strict nutritional protocol and tried to get as much healing restorative sleep as I could, and still do. I still keep away from alcohol, sugar, caffeine, MSG and aspartame most of the time. I indulge in a little dark chocolate from time to time, and make sure that I am eating non-fat products, nothing hydrogenated, all fresh dark fruits and vegetables, lots of fish, poultry (chicken and turkey) and occasionally lean pork or beef.

Each morning for breakfast I have frozen mixed berries (blueberries, raspberries and marion berries) with a few tablespoons of non-fat European style yogurt topped with flax cereal or cooked quinoa, a half a sliced banana and roasted flax seeds. I also like to add a little Splenda for sweetener. To drink with my morning vitamin supplements I make a yummy mix of four ounces prune or tomato juice with four ounces of water, add a heaping tablespoons each of ground flax and lecithin.

For lunch most days I like to have turkey, tofu or tuna on fresh dark lettuce or spinach, with raw broccoli tops and other veggies. To keep it from becoming too monotonous I add some dried cranberries and roasted flax or sunflower seeds and alternate Italian dressing with a mixture of low sodium soy sauce, flax seed oil and fresh ground pepper. I find that a nice yellow corn cracker with either garlic hummus or peanut butter with no-sugar jam on top, or an apple or banana, or low-fat cream cheese on a celery stick make great afternoon snacks. For dinner I eat a small portion of lean protein, some steamed dark vegetables and fresh veggie salad as well as my nighttime supplements. All I usually drink is filtered water or green tea. As a rule, I try to eat daily foods that are naturally high in the amino acid triptophan (that serotonin is derived from), so I often eat turkey, apples and bananas, non-fat milk products and a little dark chocolate.

My current supplement regimen consists of 960mg of malic acid with 450mg magnesium twice daily in a single magnesium malate tablet, 200mcg of selenium twice daily, 500mg of no-flush niacin twice daily, a B-100mg time release complex twice daily, 500mg of vitamin C twice daily, 1500mg of calcium with D divided twice daily, 1000iu of vitamin D daily, 400iu of vitamin E twice daily, 2400mg of soft-gel fish oil twice daily, one good multiple vitamin with minerals daily, a half of an aspirin and my daily 60mg dose of Cymbalta.

Sometimes I add to my regimen D-ribose for extra energy, but I always stick with the basic program. Nutrition has become a real adventure for me, and lots of fun. I have developed a healthy relationship between food and my emotional health and no longer use food as comfort, or eat carbohydrates or sugar for energy. The supplements you choose to meet your own specific needs may vary a little from mine, but remember to always include lots of antioxidants, calcium with D for bone strength after age forty, a high vitamin B complex for the central nervous system, and magnesium malate for muscles and soft tissue. Selenium is also important to help strengthen and maintain a strong immune system and the niacin helps open and clean the vessels to the soft tissue and extremities, helping the circulation deliver nutrients and oxygen to all the cells in the body. Niacin also helps lower cholesterol, as do lots of omega-3 essential fatty acids that are found in fish, fish oil, flax seeds, and nuts.

A strong nutritional protocol makes you feel better and stronger and helps in the healing process, a process that includes being very patient with your body as it returns to health. Although returning to health is the body's natural desire, it has to shed the unhealthy patterns that have occupied it during the duration it suffered from chronic FMS, like unlearning a very bad habit. The soft tissues, for instance, need to relearn how to function in a balanced way without remaining tight. Doing this requires letting go of old patterns that become useless and obsolete as the body heals, and periodic gentle massage can help. Never get angry at your body or at yourself.

Also, pay attention to your thoughts as you think them and keep working at choosing healthy and appropriate thoughts as much as you can. Your mind has to shed some unwanted patterns of thinking as well, so think of your mind as you would a small child who is learning how to speak. Allow the healthy thoughts to repeat themselves over and over again so they become deeply engrained into your cerebral biology and continuously reassure your mind, especially if you have experienced failed hope. Gently encourage these new thoughts as they develop neural -pathways and they will eventually become natural and easy to think. Always acknowledge and honor the messages that come from your gut instincts, your body intelligence, and do not allow inner conflicts.

Be true to yourself, trust and honor your intuition, your inner guide. Be like the old monk who chose to forge a new pathway up the other side of the mountain and remember to appreciate the view as you go. Go where there is no path and create a trail. Actively nurturing your mind and body back to health is a very self-enriching thing to do that will empower you to guide yourself confidently and persistently. Adults reassure themselves and you will need this self-assurance when you come up against the naysayers and the skeptics, not to mention the doctors in the medical profession who do not fully understand the nature of chronic fibromyalgia and have formed very strong, and potentially destructive, opinions about this condition.

An excellent example of such a doctor is a conversation about FMS I had with an eye doctor who was caring for an elderly friend. The conversation went like this:

Dr.: "What you must understand about FMS is 50% of people who claim to have it are nuts, and crazy people make it hard for doctors to treat people who actually have FMS because they can not tell them apart. The problem is they all get thrown into the same pot."

Me: "Where do you get your belief that 50% of people with FMS are crazy?"

Dr.: "I see it all the time. People come in here claiming they have FMS when they are simply crazy and there is nothing you can do to treat them. They say their vision is blurry or they get headaches because they read on the Internet that these are FMS symptoms and in reality there is nothing wrong with their eyes."

Me: "Well if you are at all interested in knowing the cause of FMS, it is being acknowledged more and more that cervical myopathy, namely the traumatic misalignment of the Atlas, causes the over-firing and hyper-sensitization of the central nervous system and accounts for the vast assortment of FMS symptoms. Are you open to alternative treatments at all?"

Dr.: "Yeah, sure I am, but patients come in here all the time that had Rolfing, deep massage and acupuncture and some have even had adjustments on their neck for months and it didn't do a thing to help them."

Me: "Did they have daily adjustment to their neck and Atlas?"

Dr.: Shaking his head vigorously, "They had months and months and it did nothing, no help at all."

Me: "Maybe they didn't have the Atlas alignment done correctly. There are many ways the Atlas can be misaligned. How many patients are you talking about?"

Dr.: "About ten. But what you are not hearing is the all important point that half of these people are crazy, and treatment does not work on crazy people and it is impossible to distinguish them from the people who really have FMS."

Me: "Well you can't disregard the results that have been made with the Atlas alignment protocol done by a chiropractor at the Fibromyalgia Relief Center in South Lake Tahoe. The results are 95% of his patients that come in with chronic FMS are cured."

Dr.: "Oh yes I can. These are testimonials and they do not count. Tell me where he's been published."

Me: "This doctor has written and published a book on the success of his protocol that just came out last year and is working on studies to be published as soon as he can, but he spends the majority of his time treating patients and getting the word out."

Dr.: "He may have written a book but it's not even valid unless he is published."

Me: "Are you are talking about being published in a medical journal with findings from a double-blind study?"

Dr.: "Absolutely! It has to be approved and validated by someone else or I won't even consider it. There are lots of quacks that claim their treatment works, but these are merely testimonials that don't count in the medical profession."

Me: "But you can't ignore results, not mine or all the people that have been cured by this protocol, and aren't you doing the same thing you complained about earlier by throwing all the alternative treatments into one pot?"

Dr.: Shaking his head no said, "Again, a treatment is only valid when there has been a double-blind study and the results are published in a credible medical journal."

Me: "Then the medical profession is shutting out an effective treatment because you can not do a double-blind study on an Atlas adjustment. You can't fake an adjustment to the neck."

Dr.: "Yes you can. There have been lots of treatments that people said a double-blind study could not be done and they found a way. Look, I am open to alternative treatments, but you are still missing the importance of what I said earlier that 50% of these patients are nuts."

Me: "Whether I agree with you on this or not, there is no known treatment in regular medicine that can help FMS anyway. Drugs only make the condition worse overall and do nothing to improve it."

Dr.: "You are assuming I am only talking about medicine. I am talking about all forms of treatment, including alternative treatments."

Me: "OK, let met rephrase. Aside from drugs, all forms of treatment will make FMS worse for a short time before benefits are gained because the body is struggling so hard to do a balancing act to keep itself alive that any form of outside stimuli will upset the balance and aggravate the FMS temporarily because the disease lives inside the central nervous system."

Dr.: "OK, yes, but an Atlas misalignment could not be the cause for all the symptoms that appear all over the body. There is not one cause for FMS. It is a tangled mess of factors and no one can untangle it."

Me: "Yes, FMS has a huge list of symptoms that involve the entire body and not all patients exhibit the same combination of symptoms, but they can all be caused by a misalignment in the Atlas because it puts torque on the meningies and a kink in the spinal cord that causes the entire spine to over-fire distortion signals into the entire body."

Dr.: "Well until I see it published its just another cracker-jack theory with no proof."

Me: "Actually if you go online to www.stopfibro.com and read all about the Atlas alignment protocol done by Dr. Whitcomb in South Lake Tahoe, you can watch hundreds of taped testimonials he does on his patients before and after the treatment and you can see his success in their faces, hear it in their voices and in how they speak."

Dr.: "Now that's the problem right there. Nutty people go online and read about it and decide they've got it when diagnosing FMS is actually a process of exclusion. After all the tests, when no other diagnosis fits, then doctors diagnose FMS."

Me: "Well actually there is a tender-point test that can be done that is currently considered the gold standard for diagnosing FMS when a patient has at least 11 out of a possible 18 tender points along with other symptoms, but do check out the website I mentioned before."

Dr.: "OK I will, but unless this guy is published I can still easily dismiss him."

Me: "As I said he has written a book that has been published (as he shook his head no) and he hasn't had the time yet to publish any other form of study because he's been so busy curing people, however he told me himself he intends to do so. Because people with FMS suffer so horrifically he's been devoting his time to treating them, and getting his book out to spread the word, and I agree with this. It would be immoral to try to trick a FMS sufferer somehow into believing they are getting an Atlas adjustment, which couldn't be done anyway, when they are suffering so unimaginably. I for one know this treatment works because I was bedridden for two years and then housebound ten years and now in the final stages of this curative treatment I am writing a book to help others find their way."

Dr.: "Well you have to believe it because you get to write a book!

With that slight, he then turned his back on me. I was stirred by the conversation, but remained calm and matter of fact in my rebuttals to his retorts. I wondered if after our conversation he concluded that I was yet another crazy person who once saw something about FMS on the Internet and thought she had it. This might account for his attempting to insult me at the end.

I saw this conversation as a gift because it presented me with the opportunity to articulate for you the opinions and thinking representing a common mindset held by many doctors in today's medical profession. While I was recounting the words on paper that had passed between the two of us, it was hard not to laugh out loud occasionally. The whole thing struck me as really being quite humorous. I understand that doctors are human and that everyone has their issues, but not everyone exerts them as an affront. The moral of this story: do not be discouraged or swayed by a few doctor's uninformed opinions and conclusions. Allow for the fact that the medical profession and the scientific community is still in the process of learning about FMS and many other chronic diseases and needs a bit more time. Meanwhile, get on with the business of taking your life back. We need not wait for them to catch up before taking matters into our own hands.

Go ahead and take action no matter what the medical profession tells you. You do not need their approval or endorsement to find your own healing combination. People sometimes tend to give medical doctors too much power over their health and well-being, or what is even worse, they give doctors absolute power. Remember that doctors are fallible human beings working in a profession for hire. You hire them from time to time for consultation and helpful advice, and like any other advice you pay for, you can either take it or not. Like anyone else, medical doctors are not always right. Taking their opinion as gospel can be disastrous in chronic fibromyalgia in these current times. So far the standard multiple drug therapy for FMS offered by the medical profession most likely will not help you feel better.

Speaking of drugs, in 2007 the FDA approved what was called "the only drug designed to effectively treat fibromyalgia." In a newspaper article in October of 2007, Lynne Matallana, co-founder of the National Fibromyalgia Association, briefly talks about her own experience with FMS. She states that she saw 37 doctors in two years before she was properly diagnosed. This type of quest gets labeled "doctor shopping" under diagnostic criteria for hypochondriasis, a stigma some doctors ignorantly attach to FMS patients. The article also talks about a drug that had been recently approved by the FDA called Lyrica created by Pfizer (one of the largest drug companies in the U.S.) made especially for "managing the pain" of FMS. There was nothing mentioned in the article about its success rate or side effects, and the drug is too young to assess the effects of long-term usage.

I do know just prior to the release of this drug I saw a battery of national TV commercials paid for by Pfizer showing tearful, depressed people who were clearly suffering from chronic pain, giving a website to "find out more about how to relieve symptoms of fibromyalgia" stating FMS is indeed a real condition. The website was designed to be educational and to introduce their new drug, however there was no mention of any drug in the TV commercial.

The address given was www.fibrohope.org and I reviewed it soon after I saw the commercial to see what was up. I am already of the opinion that drug companies can sometimes seem like bottom feeders and seek to profit from what they perceive as a "cash-cow condition." The 100+ million reported fibromyalgia patients worldwide can live their entire life seeing doctors on a regular basis, repeating expensive tests and taking a battery of expensive drugs traditionally prescribed as ongoing symptom management therapy for the rest of their lives. It is easy to see how the drug companies can view these patients as their newest cash cow. This may seem cynical, but when you compare the cost of the same drug in the U.S. to what it costs in Canada for example, the staggering U.S. mark-up leads one to naturally doubt the scruples of the drug companies in the U.S. and those of their CEOs. This is only my opinion of course.

Furthermore, the Pfizer website talked about fibromyalgia in a general way, mentioning a few ways to help yourself feel better that are well accepted such as lowering stress, eating right, getting more sleep and doing low impact exercise. Then after they discuss these generalities, they make the statement on the very last page of their promo saying, "There is no known cause for chronic FMS and no cure." They do not say "no known cure." However they do say the pain can be managed with their new drug Lyrica, "the only FDA approved drug made especially for fibromyalgia." Then they went into a long list of possible side effects that closely resembled many full-blown FMS symptoms.

It was astonishing to me that a website set up by one of largest drug companies in the U.S. called "fibrohope" would completely dash your hopes and tell you that there is no cure. In addition it is very sneaky to me that this nationwide TV campaign launched by Pfizer intending to lure in FMS sufferers with the promise of "hope," offering a toll free number for a free information kit and a website to find out more, would make no mention of what they are trying to sell.

The TV ad comes across as compassionate and benevolent as though the drug company is offering some free help to FMS sufferers, but in the end is just another "come on" to sell something aimed at people who are suffering in an inexplicable way. This looks to me like an attempt to profit off the pain, suffering, and desperation of the chronically ill, and is why I feel that drug companies can sometimes seem unscrupulous by looking to make huge profits over and above their research cost off of the illnesses the medical profession cannot cure, understand or explain.

While it is true that some drugs can help manage conditions such as hypertension and save lives at times of emergency, drug companies do not address curing chronic conditions. Nor do they encourage people to explore alternatives to the chemicals they want them to put into their body before resorting to taking them. Furthermore, they spend millions of dollars on ads designed to scare you into asking your doctor about a drug for a condition you may or may not have or get in the future, turning your doctor into a sort of front door drug dealer.

Drug companies also use media venues to brainwash society into believing the only way to live a healthier life is to take their drugs and adopt a drug lifestyle if you will, which is unhealthy. The only reason they tell you about the possible side effects of a drug is because the FDA forces them to, and the side effects often sound a bit like the condition the drug is treating, and something worse. The mixed side effects of multiple drugs can even be very dangerous. If you have more than one doctor prescribing drugs to you, be sure to have them talk to each other so no harm can come to you.

As consumers of our modern day medical profession, with all the drugs our doctors can prescribe being peddled to them by smart looking salespeople on a daily basis who constantly provide them with bags and bags of free drug samples, it is especially important for fibromyalgia patients to remember to be responsible and careful consumers. It is sometimes imperative that a multiple drug management therapy should not be resorted to if at all possible. Symptom management drugs given to FMS patients should only be used on a short-term basis and only as a last resort for chronic pain management because of the side effects. More importantly they do nothing to cure the overall condition and often make you feel worse. When the side effects of a drug or drugs are causing as many problems as the condition they are claiming to help, it makes no sense to take them.

No matter how desperate you feel about the pain levels you are experiencing with fibromyalgia, pause and read the side effects of any drug you are considering trying and the long-term effects as well. Even the strongest painkillers often only take the edge off the pain of FMS and do not "kill" the pain anyway. In addition, as your resistance to a drug increases, the dosage also increases in order to get the same initial response and eventually even the highest dosage will not work as promised, and a stronger drug will be needed. It is a very bad road to travel and can only lead to addiction, despair and hopelessness. Take it from one who has been there, done that, with the T-shirt to prove it.

Special Notes to the Reader

This book has been written from my true experience that has been an educated one, rather than an education that has never been truly experienced. My cure for FMS comes from the experience of what has worked for me. I am not a doctor, nor am I trying to practice medicine without a license. I am merely sharing what I have discovered to be true from my success in curing FMS, and showing you how to experience yours. Albert Einstein said, "True knowledge only comes through experience."

Throughout this book I talk to you in semi-depth about the many important things I have come to know as truth from experiences that have been enhanced with education. I discuss the importance of eliminating all forms of unnecessary psychological stress to heal the central nervous system, as stress makes all physical conditions worse. I have shared my personal experience in distancing myself from people, who through their dysfunctional behaviors, became detrimental to my healing, and how this led me to the ultimate truth that God, our Creator, is our true father/ mother and my family of choice can be made up of like-minded people who are safe.

I share how I am now able to experience the profound sense of psychological peace and freedom that comes from being true to myself, "living in loving detachment," and authentically forgiving all who have been harmful and unsafe to me physically and psychologically. I practice daily to maintain a healthy level of understanding, compassion and forgiveness for myself and others acquired over time with the help of psychological counseling, self-education, honest reflection and hard work.

I practice remembering that everyone is doing the best they can with what they have at the time and that everyone has a right to be where they are, grow at their own rate and live life their own way. Who am I to judge how and when this should be? My only job is to protect myself from the destructive behaviors of dysfunctional people, guard my serenity, and keep myself safe and healthy.

I honestly have no interest or desire to sit in judgment over someone else's life by disagreeing with the way they choose to live. The way others choose to live is none of my business. However, I do desire to assess everyone who crosses my path for health and safety and I only pay attention to someone else's psychological health when it adversely affects me. I am not a hypocrite. I live and let live and apply what I have learned to be healthy standards in my own life.

I understand that mature healthy adults keep their own counsel, mind their own business, do not trample on the rights and freedoms and boundaries of others (their souls), treat each other with kindness and respect, and set appropriate boundaries against chronic or major offenders for self -care when needed. After all, degrees of dysfunction are common in our society and most people can relate to experiencing this phenomenon. In my opinion, the standards and morals of our society are a bit narcissistic, self-indulgent and immature, and generally speaking, human beings need to mature and evolve as a species. However, Eckhart Tolle has written about this extensively.

So, in this book I have discussed how to use healthy and appropriate internal and external boundaries to protect against those who do harm and drain your energy with their dysfunction behaviors, and people who need to judge or attack you from a place of ignorance in order to serve their own feelings. Unless you walk in another's shoes, you cannot really know what they have experienced and it is arrogant to believe you can.

I am very careful now to only get close to people who are mature enough to be kind and respectful as a rule, are capable of taking personal responsibility for their own behavior, and are able to respect the boundaries of others without feeling compelled to trample on their rights and freedoms — people who are capable of creating and employing external and internal boundaries with themselves (self-control rather than other-control), who are never intrusive or condemning, who are interested in their own spiritual growth and evolution, and who make a sincere effort to notice the influence their behavior has on others. In other words, I do not get close to people who are chronically selfish and immature. I can no longer afford to allow dysfunctional people to interfere with my sacred serenity, and I keep my distance with detached compassion and forgiveness.

I also have discussed what I have discovered to be the cause and the cure for chronic FMS with all its pain, fatigue, depression and bizarre symptomatology. I have spoken about the universal importance of choosing to eat only for energy and nutrition, and the importance of choosing to find comfort and relief through alternative treatment modalities for pain management instead of the current management therapy of multiple heavy drugs. I emphasized the need in this text for gentle low-impact exercise to regain strength, mobility, flexibility and stamina that will prevent falling into the downward spiral of deconditioning, to eventually enable your body to hold healthy alignment on its own.

I have provided my true testimony in discussing the limitations and abuses of the medical profession with regard to chronic illness, its entanglement with big drug companies and the modern-day prescription drug culture with all its side effects and pit-falls. I explained the importance of the alternative natural medicines of classical constitutional homeopathy that stimulates the body's natural healing abilities while providing energetic support, and chiropractic care for assessment and diagnosis of the cervical spine that includes Atlas alignment and spinal correction as the most essential component in the right healing combination for curing chronic FMS.

The only drug I have mentioned possibly using for treatment is a dual neurotransmitter modulator to help reverse what I call "pain signal distortion" and to relieve depression and normalize a hyper-sensitized central nervous system to help it heal. If you do not wish to remain on this drug life-long, you can eventually plan on a trial, gradually tapering off of the drug, but only after you have established a strong pattern of wellness and a healthy life-long lifestyle. Consult your doctor for the tapering off dosages and time periods for each dose. It makes sense to help yourself during this tapering off period of transition by eating lots of turkey, apples, bananas, milk, small bites of near-pure dark chocolate and other foods that are high in triptophan – the essential amino acid that stimulates the production of brain neurotransmitters serotonin and dopa-mine. The regular production of these neurotransmitters can be altered from the stress of FMS as well as all other stresses.

Throughout this book I have sought to clearly and fairly debunk the myths surrounding chronic fibromyalgia syndrome that are both destruc-tive and self-defeating if taken to heart. Most importantly I have sought to effectively empower you, the chronic FMS sufferer, to not accept de-feat, but rather to take responsibility for your health by becoming an ex-pert on your condition and being fiercely proactive by commanding the future of your treatment. I strongly suggest you write down your life sto-ry and look for traumatic single or multiple compounding injuries or stresses to your body that would have impacted your cervical spine. With some detective work you should be able to isolate and document the events leading up to the time your chronic FMS was triggered. Have your cervical spine properly x-rayed and evaluated by a chiropractor that is experienced in both diagnosing and treating Atlas subluxation and oth-er contributing types of cervical myopathy, subsequent spinal subluxation and body-wide imbalances.

Key Questions to Ask About Your Body

- When you look in the mirror, is your head slightly tilted to one side? Do your ear lobes seem uneven to ground level? Does your chin seem slightly out of alignment with the trachea at the bottom of your neck?
- Is one leg shorter than the other with achy pains in the hip of the shortened leg?
- Do you have restless leg syndrome more on one side of the body than the other?

- Do you have TMJ on the same side as the shortened leg?
- Do you have migraine headaches that begin at the top of your neck or behind the area of TMJ?
- Do you have neck tension and difficulty with neck mobility, especially at the bottom of your neck?
- Do you have spinal misalignments in the upper and mid back that cause chronic pain and spasm, especially on one side?
- Do you have 11 out of 18 tender points in the key places?

If you continually answer "yes" to the above questions it is safe to say you have an Atlas subluxation to one side that is most likely locked in a forward position, causing pain and spasm on the opposing side of the body, compensation subluxations through the spine, a foreshortened leg, and a hyper-sensitized and hyper-activated central nervous system responsible for all the vast number of FMS symptoms that stress and chronic poor posture worsens.

Also, I want you all to do some serious soul-searching with the intention of connecting with your inner guide, your gut instinct, your natural intuition, your body intelligence, your God-self or whatever you feel comfortable calling the innate inner wisdom that exists within us all, and choose to trust it. Doing so will get you on the right path that will enable you to regain your health and take back your life. You already possess all the answers and know all that you need to know. You just need enlightenment.

Choosing to always listen to your inner wisdom, especially during times of chaos, is what I like to call "inter-netting" with God (refer to my non-religious description of the term "God" at the beginning of this book – as we all have our own idea of a higher power). If you choose to do this you cannot go wrong. My choice to trust my innate inner wisdom through critical and chaotic times has enabled me to accept or reject what was right or not right for me, and is the reason I am well today. It is the inspiration that has written this book.

Now each day seems like a kind of miracle to me. To wake up looking forward to what the day has in store, to feel comfortable in my body again – maybe even for the first time in my life, to have a relatively calm and clear mind with no real worries, and to be able to feel my joy every day and express it, all seems miraculous. No more sharp nerve pain all over my entire body, no more knots in my neck and shoulders and back, no more restless legs or body at night, no more migraine headaches, no more stomach and digestive problems (unless I indulge in too much dark chocolate or spicy food – duh!), no more brain fog (fibro-fog) or fatigue or depression. I only experience normal tiredness when I miss my afternoon nap or after having stayed up too late the night before. No more painful flare-ups, only normal soreness when I work out a bit too much. I finally feel like everybody else my age that is relatively healthy, maybe even a little better. It is amazing to me that all of the chronic symptoms I lived with, so very ill for so many years, are now becoming a distant memory in a past that is no longer real. This is what I want for you.

I think of the people with detached compassion who could not understand me and tried to do me psychological harm because my choices confronted them with their limitations. I have let them go and leave them to their lives with my blessings and forgiveness because life is too short to allow the limitations of others to adversely affect my peace of mind.

With regard to the content of this book, I do not know if I have presented enough evidence to convince the skeptics or the people whom the truths I have discovered has threatened, but this could not be more unimportant to me. I have healed myself of what is considered an incurable, degenerative, life-shortening disease that would continue to plague me for the rest of my life. I have won. I have triumphed over what appeared at one time to be insurmountable odds with the love and support of my wonderful family and devoted friends. All that matters now is the quality of my day and all the days to come.

I love life the way it really is, with my husband, my wonderful step-children who have given me so much joy, my dear mother who has become my best friend, my pets who exhale unconditional love – especially my African Gray parrot, Mozart, and all his knowing talking, my darling rescued dog, Pepper, who is a constant source of affection, and all my wonderful friends. I still work part-time in my medical billing and appeals business out of my home helping people with their insurance troubles. I do not wish to go back to working full-time right now. I was very ill for a very long time and I want to give my central nervous system and my body plenty of time to establish itself in its newly forming pattern of wellness. I do not want the stress and pressure of too many time commitments and a heavy work load. Working on this book for several hours each day on top of my part-time business has been just right.

It is time for me to be semi-retired after a life of hard work, accomplishments and struggles and take time to enjoy and appreciate all my blessings. I also want to help promote this book so I can get my story of hope to chronic FMS sufferers everywhere. All I need to do is keep believing in myself and trying my best to do what is right for me so I can preserve and continue to enhance my health. My biggest desire is to help others find their way through the long, dark tunnel of this horrific disease by shining a light bright enough for them to see their way clear to the end and back out into life again.

So I say to you all: choose to have faith in the feelings you receive from deep within your core, and pay close and equal attention to both your body and mind intelligence so you can be internally aligned and be your own teacher. Choose to be a free agent in the universe by always guiding your own life and keeping it going in forward motion, unfettered by the negativity and ignorance of others, no matter what. Choose to plug into your inner strength through the power of fact-based positive thinking and feel the hope and positive energy it generates.

Choose to burn your old map of life and create a new one by breaking old patterns and finding new ways of seeing, perceiving, thinking and being. Choose to master your own mind and correct the errors by educating yourself, selecting your thoughts wisely and forging a new path to the top of the other side of the mountain. Ralph Waldo Emerson wrote, "Do not go where the path might lead, go instead where there is no path and leave a trail." Keep in mind the limitations of allopathic (regular medicine) treatments and literally make sure your head is on straight. You have nothing to lose but your illness.

Above all, take personal responsibility, not only for mind and your behavior, but also for your body and soul, and realize you are on a serious and all-important journey of spiritual evolution as you go about the vital business of healing your body. Become an expert on your condition and on your own state of mind and remember that half-understanding is worse than ignorance. This is not merely a physical journey. You are in the midst of a complete metamorphosis from which you will emerge a newer and better version of yourself. Do not wait to get started in taking your life back! Start choosing what works to heal chronic fibromyalgia syndrome now! Find the right healing combination and "Feel the fear and do it anyway!"

I have a three-minute + digital patient story online created by Pip Hardy and Tony Sumner, founders of the Patient Voices Program and co-owners and directors of Pilgrim Projects, Cambridge, England, and winner of the 2010 international 'BMJ Award for Excellence in Healthcare Education.' The stories from the Patient Voices Program are used in Royal colleges and Universities globally. To view it, go to my website at www.thefibrocure.com. It was beautifully created and includes a narrative of my voice telling my story over selected pictures that show my progress from illness to regaining my health and taking back my life. I hope you will enjoy it.

I'd like to give special thanks to my devoted and very talented upper cervical chiropractor, Dr. Peter Ruiz of Monterey, CA for his help to me over the past few years. His care has been a major factor in my regaining a state of health and well-being. Without it, maintaining my cure and remaining FMS free would not have been possible.

My Protocol for a Lasting Cure — What worked for me

Find a reputable upper cervical chiropractor that can x-ray down your throat for an Atlas subluxation and evaluate your neck and spine for subsequent compensation subluxations. Make sure this doctor has the experience and expertise to provide the necessary treatment for creating healthy alignment of your neck and spine and has experience in helping people with FMS. It would be best if he or she had the special table called the Atlas alignment "Side Posture Head Drop Table" originally invented by Dr. B. J. Palmer, DC who is the founder of the method.

One brand is called the "Nicholas Brand" among others. If there is a left or right shift in your Atlas, it is most likely locked in forward position, along with a head tilt. This subluxation will need this type of head drop table adjustment to unlock it. Once your ligaments become strong enough to hold the Atlas in a "locked down" position, the rest of your spine will go through a few changes to realign itself with the head being back "on point" with the center of gravity. Your entire body will need to "decompensate" from the period of time the Atlas was out of alignment. Hang in there, stick with it and be patient.

Find a reputable, licensed homeopath that specializes in classical, constitutional homeopathy. A good homeopath can match you to the correct constitutional remedy in one to three tries. If they cannot succeed in matching you after four tries, change to another homeopath. Classic constitutional homeopathy will initiate a deep healing response and provide good energetic support while you are experiencing the ups and downs of healing. A healing course of treatment may last as long as two to ten years depending on the severity and length of your illness, however it is very inexpensive and you only need to see your homeopath for thirty minute follow-up interviews every three or four months after your initial two hour interview. Again, hang in there, stick with it and be patient.

To locate a classical homeopath in your area, contact The American Institute of Homeopathy at: 101 S. Whiting St. #16, Alexandria, VA, or go online to http://www.arizonahomeopathic.org, or write to P.O. Box 38284 Phoenix, AZ, 85069-8183, or call (602) 263-3589. You may need to travel a little bit to get to one, but since you only will need to see them once every three months or so at the start, then less as time goes by, it would be worth it for sure. I meet with my homeopath once every 4 ½ months, and travel 60 minutes one way to see her every other visit, alternating physical visits with visits over the phone. This has worked out for us both beautifully.

Find a reputable psychotherapist or psychologist and utilize this care provider in a goal oriented way up to two years. Be sure to use this course of treatment to facilitate "process efficiency" and help you build a bridge over the deep waters of transformation as you process yourself out of the past into the present through guided, goal-oriented education. Do not use this service provider as a crutch. As you take back your life, a good therapist will support you, and teach you the skills you need to live your life in a healthier, safer and more prosperous way. Be sure he or she understands your condition. Work at it, be gentle with yourself, and it will soon begin working for you.

Initiate a comprehensive nutritional protocol within reason and make it a permanent part of your life. Consider this new protocol as a "live-it" rather than a "die-it" and commit yourself entirely to a nutritional lifestyle. This will provide your body with the tools necessary to naturally repair and heal your biology from the ravages of chronic FMS. Remember that a comprehensive nutritional protocol includes nutritional supplements, eating all the right foods and rarely eating all the wrong ones. Your body wants to be well and wants to heal itself. Cooperate with it and give it the tools it needs to build a new pattern of wellness throughout your entire body all the way down to the cellular level. Cherish your body as the temple of your soul.

Begin moving and gently exercising at a level that will not set you back or flare you up too much. Begin light and easy, pick a form of exercise that seems enjoyable to you and build slowly from there. Never, ever push or try to build too quickly. As you gain strength, flexibility and stamina, you can gently step up your game. Remember to concentrate on your breathing and if it gets labored a bit, ease off. Exercising needs to become a permanent part of your life to reverse deconditioning and maintain strength and flexibility. Remember that it takes a long time to recondition a body that has become out-of-shape or atrophied. A physical therapist once told me that it takes approximately 2,200 movements of a muscle in a state of atrophy to bring it back into a state of healthy conditioning. As always, stick with it, go slow and be patient.

Use natural alternative pain management therapies that are gentle and easy. Pick one that appeals to you, and do not try more than one modality at a time, otherwise you will not be able to tell what is helping and what is not. Give it a month or two and if you are not feeling better, move on to another option. Remember that no matter what a caregiver says, make sure they understand your condition and know to go easy on you. Also make sure that they have had success helping other FMS patients with their method and do not expect you to stick with it if you do not feel it is helping in a reasonable time frame.

Eliminate all unnecessary stresses from your life by making the necessary changes. Make those tough choices, set those boundaries and make your health the number one priority over any and all relationships in your life. Do not waste your limited, precious time and energy trying to educate others or explain your reasons to "make them understand" who may not possess the capability or capacity. Demand respect and do not allow anyone to judge or demean you, or intrude on your serenity. You have every right to do whatever is necessary to recover your health. Do not waste one ounce of healing energy on guilt, shame or false obligation. Your first responsibility is to yourself and you deserve a chance to take back your life from this monster illness, and live it again in health, peace and prosperity! This is your new mindset for life!

Getting Your Insurance to Pay, Proving Medical Necessity

I felt I could prove medical necessity if I used my chiropractor's first, more conservative, treatment plan as a starting point from which to justify the need for a second, more aggressive, treatment plan. I felt by contrasting the limited results from the first plan with the dramatic results from second, medical necessity would become apparent. Based on the success of the second treatment plan this strategy worked beautifully.

When my first denial came through, I naturally had to go through the claims appeals and hearing process as well as arrange a conference call between my chiropractor, a requested doctor of his peers (another chiropractor serving on the hearing board) and me. The insurance company's representative was so highly impressed with my knowledge and the success from the more aggressive treatment plan he approved all my treatments – past, present and future. He even asked for a copy of this book!

I was easily able to contrast the results from the first treatment plan with those of the second and show how the second plan had worked well in improving my condition and dramatically increasing my activities of daily living. It pays to believe in yourself, follow through to the extent of your rights, and not give up at your first or second denial. Also, it pays to follow your instincts and not listen to the critics and skeptics. There is an old joke about "The birth of the artist, and the afterbirth; the critic," that applies here. So be the artist, create a new path, take independent action and never mind the bad reviews.

Eight Steps to Getting Your Chiropractic Treatment Covered by Insurance

1) First check your policy to see if it has a benefit provision for chiropractic care. If there is no benefit provision for chiropractic then the subject becomes moot. However these days most insurance companies cover it because chiropractors are the second largest medical provider group used next to physicians.

2) Check to see if the provision has a "guideline" or a "limit" that restricts benefits. A limit is usually ironclad, however a guideline is subject to certain conditions, such as medical necessity. A limit can sometimes be subject to medical necessity, but not always.

3) If your benefit provision has a "guideline" it will either be for coverage up to a certain number of visits per year or per condition, unless further treatment is proven to be medically necessary. If proven, then benefits can be extended according to your doctor's recommendations and the discretion of the insurance company.

4) Start by having your chiropractor bill your insurance for each visit as you see him or her. Be sure to have the doctor's office include your FMS diagnosis with any other malady that has been detected by him or her on all claims and letters.

5) As soon as your insurance first denies a visit due to a policy maximum benefit, make a copy of the denial, a copy of your doctor's itemized billings and resubmit it to your insurance company with a letter of medical necessity from your chiropractor. Include a cover letter requesting your claim be reviewed and paid on the basis of medical necessity. Conclude your letter with the statement: "I intend to pursue this matter to fullest extent of my rights," and ask for a written response to this review. Keep a duplicate of all correspondence with your insurance.

6) If the reviewed claim comes back denied, then get second letter of medical necessity for chiropractic care from your general physician including your diagnosis of FMS. Resubmit the claim with the second letter along with copies of all previous documents and write a cover letter yourself requesting a second review with an independent review board. In your letter, tell the insurance how limited your activities of daily living (ADLs) were at the onset of your treatment and how much they have improved as a result of your treatment. Describe these initial limits to your

ADLs and the improvements in detail. Note: Sometimes an insurance company will only re-review up to two or three times depending on the cost and availability of independent reviewers.

7) Then, if the second review is denied, resubmit the entire review package again along with all of the visits to date to the insurance company and this time ask for a "fair hearing" with a hearing board that has at least one chiropractor on it. Your chiropractor will refer to this as "a doctor of his peers." Call your insurance and get the name and address of the person in charge of scheduling hearings and address your package to their attention. This will become your contact person. Always ask for a written response.

8) If the results of the hearing are unfavorable, then call your contact person and request a second hearing, this time in the form of a three-way phone consultation between yourself, your chiropractor and chiropractor from the hearing board. Coordinate this consultation with the insurance's chiropractor, your chiropractor, and yourself in the form of an appointment in your chiropractor's office. When the consultation takes place allow the doctors to speak first and then be ready to talk to the insurance doctor personally and answer his or her questions. Be sure to assert yourself and how much your FMS has improved due to the care you have received from your chiropractor in light of your ADLs and overall health. It is very important to speak to them personally.

This may seem like an arduous task, but when you are having multiple treatments over a period of time, it will help your overall sense of calm and well-being if you know your treatments will continue to be covered until you have recovered your health and beyond. Insurance companies routinely put their customers through this process hoping they will tire of it, give up and drop out. Do not let this upset you, frustrate you or make you angry. They all try to save paying out benefits whenever they can and the use of a "guideline" subject to medical necessity is the most innocuous way they can meet this goal without appearing too obvious. Simply view this process as a small job on the side to save money and earn benefits. It is worth exerting a little effort for.

Final Tips to Remember

Remember, FMS is a symptom of the Atlas subluxation (misalignment) that causes a brain stem injury that hyper-activates and hyper-sensitizes the central nervous system, and over time creates all fibromyalgia symptoms. This subluxation injury can be caused by all kinds of traumas. The most frequent cause is whiplash from an auto accident.

Consider that in the U.S. more than four million people are injured in auto accidents each year. These injuries often go unreported, and what's worse, the lower impact injuries go untreated! These are the low-impact collisions, and are the ones that will usually cause the most damage over time due to lack of immediate pain and resulting neglect. It has been established that impacts between speeds of eight to twenty M.P.H. create a G force exerted on the head and neck of over eleven G, which will result in a brain stem injury in over half of these victims.

Bumps from fender benders or rear end collisions have a very serious effect on the body because they cause misalignments (subluxations) in the spinal vertebrae that may not cause pain right away. Stiffness may be the only immediate symptoms. However, over time these misalignments can cause devastating degenerative affects to the vertebrae, the discs, the nerves in the involved areas, and the entire central nervous system resulting in chronic fibromyalgia syndrome.

Other kinds of head and neck traumas that can cause the Atlas subluxation and resulting brain stem injury are; a fall and bump on the head; a lifting while twisting accident; chronic poor head posture; general anesthesia that relaxes the neck muscles so much that the Atlas slips out if the head and neck are not supported properly during a procedure; an improperly executed golf swing; suddenly twisting the head and neck too far; and even lifting heavy babies!

This is why any and all traumas to the head and neck and spine must immediately be checked out by a qualified cervical spine chiropractor. There is a special x-ray down the throat that can be done to assess the alignment of the Atlas vertebra in particular, and regular x-rays of the neck and spine can detect any compensative subluxations that an Atlas misalignment can create throughout the spine. These subluxations can be corrected over time.

There is also a special "Atlas side posture head drop table" that is the most effective way to correct an Atlas subluxation because it is specifically designed for unlocking a forward shift and accurately aligning the Atlas. Combining chiropractic alignment of the Atlas and spine with the other legitimate alternative therapies in my protocol for a cure—what worked for me—will rehabilitate the body and central nervous system, bringing them back into balance and a state of health.

Remember, since the Atlas subluxation distorts the signals coming from and into the brain impairing brain function, the brain needs rehabilitation also. Nutrition for brain health is very important to restore the proper functioning of the organs of the brain and the production of neurotransmitters. Neurotransmitters are the chemicals that send messages between the nerves in the brain and body. They are very sensitive to the nutrients that are circulating in the body and when they are out of balance you can feel increased depression and pain.

This means eating right is crucial, and beginning the day with a breakfast of protein and wholesome carbohydrates can become your main meal of the day, and eat light at lunch and dinner. Select lower sugar fruits like berries, apples and kiwi that are fresh or frozen if not in season. Whole grain bread and cereals are the best. A breakfast of eggs, fruit and whole grain bread will boost your metabolism and even out how you feel during the day.

Proteins provide many of the building blocks for the production of neurotransmitters and should be included in all your meals. Good sources are fish, poultry that are not deep fried, eggs, cheese, soy and nuts. Low starch/high fiber vegetables like spinach, kale, tomatoes, asparagus, cucumber, carrots and cauliflower are excellent sources of brain nutrients. Try to always eat fresh, or frozen if fresh is not available. Snack on these fruits and vegetables. Cook with olive oil or macadamia nut oil filled with omega-3 oleic acids, which are anti-inflammatory compounds.

Drink fluids like hot or iced green tea and chamomile tea, and plenty of water. Avoid beverages with caffeine and sugar. Although green tea has some caffeine in it, it also has L-theanine, an amino acid, which contributes to a calm feeling. Drinking Chamomile tea at night along with an occasional L-theanine tablet is a natural way to drift off into restorative sleep when you are having trouble falling to sleep.

To avoid any nutritional deficiencies, always include B-complex 100mg vitamins to your nutritional protocol. B vitamins pay an important role in neurological health, and aid the rehabilitation process of the central nervous system when curing chronic fibromyalgia. The omega-3 essential fatty acids such as fish oil should always be included as well because they play an important role in keeping your brain fit and functioning properly.

Remember that healing is always up and down, but more up than down. It is two steps forward and one step back, then three steps forward and one step back. After a while when you have gained some ground, healing is more like four steps forward and one step back, and so on. Rate of healing is different with everyone, but it always takes this same form. Rate of healing also depends upon how long a person has been ill with FMS, how serious their illness has been, the condition they were in when they got sick, the condition they are in at the time they begin the cure, and the mental attitudes they choose to maintain throughout the healing process. Do not ever allow flare-ups or setbacks to discourage you. You must always keep a positive attitude and keep going forward no matter what.

Remember just because more women get chronic fibromyalgia syndrome then men does not mean that FMS is caused by a hormonal, female or genetic factor. The scientific community and the medical profession cannot as yet give a reasonable singular explanation for this. There is an answer to this phenomenon that is so sensible and simple they miss it. Men are simply built physically stronger than woman and have stronger musculature in their necks, shoulders and backs. If they suffer a whiplash from an auto accident, a blow on the head or a lifting accident for instance, they are less vulnerable to experiencing a misalignment of their Atlas than women are who have weaker and more delicate necks. Makes perfect sense, doesn't it?

Remember to use common sense and your own knowing when you read the latest research articles and studies and their findings regarding FMS and do not allow yourself to become brainwashed or intimidated by them. The scientific community and medical profession will always come up with new theories for a possible cause of FMS as they study each symptom. Remember the scientific community and the medical profession have their hands tied in many ways and are also controlled by the American Medical Association. Furthermore, they do not include chiropractic science in their realm of investigations, so all they can really do is to continue to identify and study symptom and extrapolate theories of cause from the results of these studies.

For instance, a recent 2009 article in *Science Daily* states the latest research shows a decrease in gray matter density inside the brains of patients with chronic FMS, however the cause is unknown. Their conclusion was, "There were significant gray matter reductions in the fibromyalgia patients studied, and FMS patients showed a strong correlation of dopamine (a neurotransmitter) levels and gray matter density in parts of the brain which dopamine controls neurological activity." The author goes on to conclude that this connection between dopamine levels and gray matter density provides "novel insights to a possible mechanism that explains some of the abnormal brain morphology associated with fibromyalgia." These remarks seem to suggest this phenomenon to be a possible cause of FMS when the reverse is true.

The Journal of Neuroscience recently reported the results from a study done by the McGill University Center for research on pain that stated, "The longer the individual has had fibromyalgia, the greater the gray matter loss, with each year of fibromyalgia being equivalent to 9.5 times the loss in normal aging." These results would have you believe this loss may be enormous and that it may be permanent. I was very ill for thirteen years and many of them were spent in the fog of fibromyalgia cognitive impairment. I struggled through 40+ books and researched countless articles, sometimes having to read them more than once to absorb them to any meaningful degree. Then I began to write the main body of this book while I was still sick, always knowing by the time I was well my book would be finished and my brain would be back to normal. It all came true, proving that no symptom of FMS is irreversible with the exception of physical damage that causes restricted movement.

I have already addressed reduction in gray matter density under theories of psychological causes in the section on stress. Science has long since verified chronic stress causes a chronic fight or flight response creating a continuous production of the "death hormones" cortisol and adrenaline. When these circulate throughout the body and brain continuously, they have devastating effects. One of which is the shrinking of gray matter in the brain and another is interference in the regular production of neurotransmitters serotonin and dopamine. As you know, the "fight or flight" response people with FMS commonly live with 24/7 year after year is exactly the kind of stress that causes this phenomenon to occur. Relieving FMS stress from the body will stop this occurrence and give the brain the chance to heal itself and return to normal functioning. Bear in mind science cannot always connect all of its own dots in order to see the big picture, neither can it measure or factor in common sense.

So if your doctor says your dopamine levels may be low due to possible decreased gray matter, eat lots of foods like turkey, bananas, apples, milk and small amounts of 85% dark chocolate daily. These foods all contain high levels of triptophan that raises the level of serotonin and dopamine production naturally. So do not get this symptom mixed up with the cause. By all means, keep reading these articles when they come along if you would like, but remember to process these articles with good old common sense and what you already know.

Remember if you have been ill with chronic FMS for a long time, your soft tissues have developed a very deep pattern of tension that will take time to re-educate. To break the tension habit in your soft tissues, you will need to stretch daily. Restorative yoga teaches a great many ways to do this safely. I personally recommend doing the "cat-cow" stretch for a set of repetitions each day, about ten to twenty times slowly. This teaches the spine to remain limber and supple throughout the day and lengthens and strengthens the soft tissues of your back, neck and shoulders. Follow with "child's pose" for five minutes. This rests the central nervous system and safely stretches the muscles in the upper and lower back.

Sitting cross legged for ten to twenty minutes on a soft cushion on the floor daily with your belly pulled gently into your spine will strengthen your posture muscles that support your back throughout the day and develop straight posture with the head sitting in a neutral position on top of the spine at all times. Always do the yoga breathing through your practices, breathing in and out through the nose, and forming a "so" position inside your mouth and throat on the in breath and an "ah" position on the out breath. This makes a throaty humming sound that should vibrate throughout the body and soothe the central nervous system.

Re-educating your soft tissues is a key component in maintaining your recovery, so commit to it daily, stick with it long-term, and be very gentle and patient with your body. Love your soft tissues compassionately because they have been through the same hell as you. Your body is willing to heal, to learn how to be healthy again, and to respond to the loving care you will give it from now on. Honor it and respect the opportunity to care for this temple of your soul that will carry you into a bright and meaningful future. The quality of your life and your thoughts will depend on how well you choose to behave toward your body from now on. You have possibly seen your body as a Judas thus far. It was not your body's fault this happened, nor was it yours. It just happened, and now you have the power to correct it. Be thankful.

Remember not to identify with your condition, no matter what it is. A mental or physical condition of any sort means there is something out of order. The truth is that you are not a condition, nor are you a disorder. You are a perfect healthy being beneath the disorder that has every right to emerge and actualize. Do not say "my fibromyalgia" – say "the fibromyalgia" or "the illness." Realize by rejecting any identification with an illness or a disorder, you are claiming who you truly are. Realize you must resolve yourself deeply to correcting whatever is wrong and create the order psychologically and physically that will allow you to fulfill your truest potential and live a happy and prosperous life.

Maintaining Your Recovery to Remain Fibromyalgia-Free

Maintaining your recovery is very important. As I mentioned above, soft tissues have memory, and so does the CNS. How I maintain my recovery after thirteen years of FMS is simple. I live as stress-free a lifestyle as possible, living in loving detachment from others with compassion, forgiveness and healthy internal and external boundaries, controlling my thoughts as appropriately as I can, exercising daily by power-walking one mile, swimming laps for forty-five minutes once or twice a week, going to restorative yoga classes a couple times a week, doing my favorite yoga stretching daily, eating right, following a strict nutritional protocol and getting a good night's sleep each night.

I go in for a chiropractic check-up every three to five weeks to make sure there are no subluxations occurring in my neck or spine. If I feel even the slightest tweak of an FMS symptom, it always means the Atlas has slipped slightly and stressed my neck and spine, and as soon as I get adjusted, all is well again. I also visit my homeopath every four months to monitor my overall energy through life's normal challenges, and when I need energetic support I get a re-dose of the appropriate remedy that usually lasts up to a year.

This is maximizing healthy living, even for someone who is not recovering from a chronic illness. I have maintained a full recovery for over two years now and continue to become stronger while living a normal, happy and prosperous life. So can you. Each new day for the rest of your life, you will either be making choices that create health or choices that create illness that you alone are responsible for. In the real world there is never a place you arrive at when this will not be so. This ongoing responsibility must be accepted as a natural reality for each of us. Spiritually it can be a very rewarding way to go about living one's life, with the satisfaction of knowing that you are in charge of the quality of your life, both psychologically and physically, and that this important job is not left up to someone else. The power is in your hand to choose what works to cure chronic fibromyalgia and live the best life you can.

Healthy Yardstick to Apply to Your Life and Relationships

Remember That Adults
- Keep their own counsel and make their own decisions with no need to justify or explain.
- Live and let live, mind their own business, and are not intrusive to others.
- Do not sit in judgment over others.
- Respect the sacred human rights and freedoms of others to live their lives as they see fit according to what they feel is best for them.
- Set appropriate boundaries for safety and health.
- Are aware of and take responsibility for their behavior.
- Are honest with themselves and others.
- Try to do no harm.

It is not wishful thinking to believe all of this is possible as long as you commit yourself to the hard work required to recreate yourself from the inside out, and grab the golden ring. Grabbing the golden ring is grabbing on to a bright future with the ability to handle whatever comes your way with dignity, grace and maturity and the confidence you have gained from guiding yourself back to wellness. So go for it. Reach for the golden ring. Reach for your truth. Reach for your health!

With all my very best wishes and highest hopes for your regained health, happiness and prosperity,

Valerie Lumley

End Notes

The EMDR Training Institute is located on 54 Penny Lane in Watsonville, CA 95076. Their phone number is (831) 372-3900.

4Life Transfer Factor at www.4life.com on line or you can call them directly at (866) 315-4002 to learn more.

ISAGENIX at www.support@isogenix.net.

"Prescription for Nutritional Healing," written by Phyllis A. Balch, CNC and James F. Balch, MD.

Nordic Naturals, Watsonville, CA at (800) 662-2544, or at www.nordicknaturals.com, or get more information at www.omega-research.com.

The American Institute of Homeopathy, 101 S. Whiting St. #16, Alexandria, VA, or at www.arizonahomeopathic.org, or write to P.O. Box 38284 Phoenix, AZ, 85069-8183, or call (602) 263-3589.

National Upper Cervical Chiropractic Association, Inc., 1489 West Warm Springs Rd., Ste. 110, Henderson, Nevada 89014, (800)541-5799. National Upper Cervical Chiropractic Assoc: NUCCA Email: info@nucca.org

International Chiropractor Association (ICA), Established by B.J. Palmer in 1926, 6400 Arlington Blvd. Ste. 800, Falls Church, VA 22042, Website: http://www.chiropractic.org, Email: info@chiropractic.org, Phone: (800) 423-4690, (703) 528-5000.

ICA Upper Cervical Council (2008), Council on Upper Cervical Care, 1110 North Glebe Rd., Ste. 650, Arlington, VA 22201, Website: http://uppercervicalcouncil.com, Email: uppercervical@chiropractic.org. Phone: (800) 423-4690, (703) 528-5000.

American Homeopathic and Integrative Medical Association, P.O. Box 10131, Phoenix, AZ 85064, Phone: (602)263-3589, Website: www.arizonahomeopathic.org, AHIMA Email: azhomeopath@aol.com.

BIBLIOGRAPHY

Cloud, Henry & Townsend, John. (1992). *Boundaries*. Grand Rapids, Michigan: Zondervan Publishing House.

Balch, Phyllis A, CNC & Balch, James F., MD. (2000). *Prescription for Nutritional Healing*. Fibromyalgia Syndrome. (p. 374). New York: Penguin Putnam, Inc.

Balch, Phyllis A, CNC & Balch, James F., MD. (2000) *Prescriptions for Nutritional Healing*. TMJ Syndrome. (p. 656). New York: Penguin Putnam, Inc.

From *http://www.ProHealth'sImmuneSupport.com*. The World's Largest Fibromyalgia & Chronic Fatigue Syndrome Website. Malic Acid and Fibromyalgia.

Balch, Phyllis A, CNC & Balch, James F., MD. (2000) *Prescriptions for Nutritional Healing*. Stress. (p. 646). New York: Penguin Putnam, Inc.

From *http://www.kirjasto.sci.fi/parace.htm*. Theophrastus Bombastus von Honhenheim AKA Philippus Aureolus Paracelsus.

Diagnostic Statistical Manual of Mental Disorders. (Vol. IV). Somatization Disorder Dx #300.81. (p. 466).

Diagnostic Statistical Manual of Mental Disorders. (Vol. IV). Conversion Disorder. Dx #300.11. (p. 452).

Diagnostic Statistical Manual of Mental Disorders. (Vol. IV). Pain Disorder. Dx #307.89. (p. 458).

Diagnostic Statistical Manual of Mental Disorders. (Vol. IV). Hypochondriasis. Dx #300.70. (p. 462).

James, Muriel & Jongeward, Dorothy. (1984). *Born To Win*. Philippines: Addison-Wesley Publishing Company, Inc.

From *Time Magazine-Special Issue*. (2003, Jan.) How Your Mind Can Heal Your Body.

From *Institute for Natural Resources*. (2005, June). Stress, Depression and Pain. (pp. 1-32).

Giles, L.G.F., DC, PhD & Muller, R., PhD. (July 15, 2003). *Up C Spine Magazine*. Chronic Spinal Pain: A Randomized Clinical Trial. (28 (14): pp. 1490-1502).

Macfarlane, G. J. & Mc Beth, J. & Silman, A. J. (2001, Sept. 22). Widespread Body Pain and Mortality. Prospective Population Based Study. *British Medical Journal*. (p. 323:662).

Banic, B. & Petersen-Felix, S. & Andersen, O. & Radanov, B., PM. (2004, Jan.).
Pain Magazine. Evidence for Spinal Cord Hypersensitivity in Chronic Pain After Whiplash Injury and in Fibromyalgia. (pp. 7-15).

Smith, J. & Terpening, C. & Seigfried of Schmidt and Gums. (2001, June). *The Annals of Pharmacotherapy.* Relief of Fibromyalgia Symptoms Following Discontinuation of Dietary Excitotoxins. (Vol. 35, No.6, pp. 702-706).

Omoigui, Soto, MD. (2007). *A Medical Hypothesis.* The Biochemical Origin of Pain: The Origin of all Pain is Inflammation and the Inflammation Response: Inflammatory Profile of Pain Syndrome: (Vol. 69). (pp. 1169-1178). Los Angeles, CA: The Division of Inflammation and Pain Research, Los Angeles Pain Clinic, CA.

From *Biomedical Science.* (2006). Activity Dependent Neuroplasticity. (pp. 185- 206). University of CA, Riverside.

From *Conference on Chronic Pain.* (2002, Oct.). Overview of Chronic Pain. Los Angeles, CA. (pp. 1-7).

St. Amand, R. Paul, MD & Marek, Claudia Craig. (1999) *What Your Doctor May NOT Tell You About Fibromyalgia.* New York: Warner Books.

From *Up C Spine – Evidence.* (2005). The Anatomy of the Atlas Subluxation. *http://www.upcspine.com/anatomy2.htm.* (pp. 1-9).

Hammer, Warren, MS, DC, DOBCO. (1983). The Dural Connection. From *http://www.chiroweb.com/hg/14/04.html.* (pp. 1-2).

From *Wikipedia.* (2008, Nov). Rectus Capitis Posterior Minor Muscle. (pp. 1-3).

Wood, P.B. & Ledbetter, C.R. & Glabus, M.F. & Broadwell, L.K. & Patterson, J.C. 2nd. (2009, Jan). *Pain Magazine.* Hippocampal Metabolite Abnormalities in Fibromyalgia: Correlation With Clinical Features. (10(1): pp. 47-52).

Emad, Y. & Ragob, Y. & Seinhom, F. & El-Khouly, G. & Abou-Seid, A. & Raskerm J. J. (2008, July). *J. Rheumatol.* Hippocampus Dysfunction May Explain Symptoms of Fibromyalgia Syndrome. A Study With Single-Voxel Magnetic Resonance Spectroscopy. (35 (7) pp. 1371-1377).

Eriksen, Kirk, DC (2002, Jan/Feb). *Today's Chiropractic.* The Development and Protocol of the Grostic/Orthospinology Procedure – Part 1. *http://www.todayschiropractic.com/issues/archives/ jan_feb_02/.* (pp. 1-3).

McAlpine, J.E., DC and J.K. Humber, DC. (1983, Jan/Feb). *Today's Chiropractor.* Chiropractic Orthospinology. Academy of Upper Cervical Chiropractic Organization, Inc. (pp. 24-28/53-54).

Rich Smith, Rich. *Chiropractic Products.* (2001, Sept.). Whole in the head. (pp. 14-18).

Smith, J.D. & Terpening, C.M. & Siegfried of Schmidt and J.G. Gums. (2001, June). *The Annals of Pharmacotherapy.* (Vol.35, No.6). Relief of Fibromyalgia Symptoms Following Discontinuation of Dietary Excitotoxins. (pp. 702-706).

Parachin, Victor, M. Div. (1995, May). *Delicious Magazine.* Eight Strategies For Living With A Serious Illness. (p. 34).

From *The Feldenkrais Guild of North America.* The Feldenkrais Method-HowYour Body is Meant To Be. http://*www.guild@feldenkrais.com.*

Olson, Lydia, Tai Chi Instructor. (2006, June). How Tai Chi Works. Monterey Peninsula College, Monterey, CA. (p. 1).

Lam, Paul, Dr. (2006, July). *Monterey Bay Healing Tao.* Tai Chi For Arthritis. Monterey, CA. (pp. 1-2).

Balch, Phyllis A., CNC & Balch, James F., MD. (2000). *Prescriptions for Nutritional_Healing.* Pain Control. (pp.720-731). New York: Penguin Putnam, Inc.

Balch, Phyllis A., CNC & Balch, James F., MD. *Prescriptions for Nutritional Healing.* Yoga. (pp. 732-733). New York: Penguin Putman, Inc.

From *Depression-Guide.com.* (2007, Oct). Psychotherapy or Talk Therapy. *http://www.depression-guide/phychotherapy.htm.* (pp. 1-3).

Mayo Staff. (2006, 1 Sept). *Mental Health-Mayo Clinic.com.* *http://www.mayoclinic.com/health/psychotherapy/MH00009.* Psychotherapy: An Overview of the Types of Therapy. (pp.1-4).

Thrash, Barry. (2007, 12 June). *Healthy News.* Talk Therapy Helps Borderline Personality Disorder. (pp. 1-2).

Castleman, Michael. (1006, Jan/Feb). *Natural Health.* Lifting The Veil. (pp. 96-99/134).

Powell, Cherith & Forde, Greg. (1996/July/Aug). *Natural Health.* It's All in Your Head. (pp. 48-52).

Shapiro, Francine, PhD. (1989). *Mental Research Institute, Inc. Palo Alto, CA.* EMDR-Eye Movement Desensitization and Reprocessing: A New Treatment for Post Traumatic Stress Disorder. (pp. 211-217).

Ullman, Dana, MPH. (1993). *Beginners Guide to Homeopathy.* (pp. 1-13).

Cohen, Karen, DC. *Introduction to Homeopathy.* (pp. 1-15).

Balch, Phyllis A., CNC & Balch, James F., MD. *Prescriptions for Nutritional Healing.* Homeopathy. (pp. 714-715). New York: Penguin Putman, Inc.

From *4Life Transfer Factor.* (2005). (Vol.1.011105, Item#81635). (p. 1-2).

Galland, Leo, MD. (2006). The Chemistry of Healing. Essay. (pp. 1-6).

Shils, Olson and Shikes. (1994). *Modern Nutrition in Health and Disease.* Fats. (pp. 1-5).

From *Nutritional News.* (1995, Dec). Malic Acid and Fibromyalgia. (pp. 1-2).

Baylock, Russel, MD. (1997). *Health Press.* Excitotoxins. The Taste That Kills.

Schwartz, George. (1999). *Health Press.* In Bad Taste. The MSG Symptoms Complex.

From http://www.jedisaber.com/DarkAngle/ency/triptophan.htm. (2005, June). Triptophan. (pp. 1-2).

From *Fibromyalgia Relief Center.* (2009, Mar). Nutrition and Diet Therapy. (pp. 1-3)

Cohen, Karen, DC. (2007). *Branciforte Chiropractic.* Cholesterol Reduction. (pp. 1-3).

From *Nutritional News.* (1995, Dec). Malic Acid and Fibromyalgia. (pp. 1-2).

Oz, Mehmet & Roizen, Michael. (2009, May). *Esquire.* The Better Man. (pp. 55-58).

Zeliger, Bernard, DO. (2008, Sept). *College of Orthopedic Medicine.* Non-Surgical Spinal Decompression. (pp. 1-3).

Guenette, Christial, DC. (2009, Oct). *Topic of the Week.* Vitamin D – Another Option to Fight Flu. (pp. 1-2).

Boswell, Mark & Cole, B. Eliot. (2006). *American Academy of Pain Management.* Weiner's Pain Management-A Protocol for Clinicians. (p 1).

Prescott, Susan & Calder, Philip. (2004, Mar). N-3 Polyunsaturated Fatty Acids and Allergic Disease. *Current Opinion in Clinical Nutrition and Metabolic Care.* (Vol. 7(2)). (pp. 123-129).

Marmorstein, Stuart, Dr. (2009, Nov). Bio-Cranial Therapy-What is the Technique? (p. 1).

Simopoulos, Artemis P., MD. (2007, July). *The Center for Genetics, Nutrition and Health, Washing, DC.* Omega-3 Fatty Acids and Athletics-Current Sports Medicine Reposts. (pp. 1-6).

Farley, Kennety. (1987, June). Karma Explained. Portions from Farley's TV show. http://wwwourworld.compuserve.com/homepage/kenneth_hirst/KarmaExp.htm.(pp. 1-4).

Khalsa, Karta Purkh Singh, DN-C, RN. (2006, Oct). *Alternative Medicine Magazine.* Confronting Fibromyalgia. (pp. 65-59).

National Fibromyalgia Association. (2007, Oct). Coping Better With Fibromyalgia with Lyrica from Pfizer Drugs. From http:www.fibrohope.org.

American Academy of Pain Management (AAPM). (2006) *Practical Guide for Clinicians, 7th Edition.* (pp. 584-585).

From Achives of Internal Medicine. (2009). *Long term effects of a very low-carbohydrate and a low-fat diet on mood and cognitive function.* Pp. 169 (20); 1873-1880).

About the Author

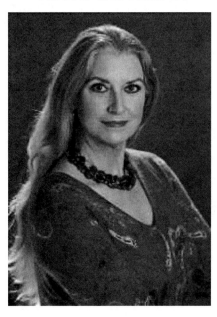

Valerie Lumley is a recovered fibromyalgic who had to leave the care of the medical profession to discover the cause and a cure for chronic fibromyalgia syndrome (FMS) in alternative medical care. Her protocol for a lasting cure is maintainable and real, and does not include a long list of addictive pharmaceuticals. It includes one prescription (a dual neurotransmitter reuptake inhibitor for normalizing the hyper-sensitized central nervous system caused by FMS) and the rest is holistic, naturopathic and non-invasive. This protocol puts the power to cure this miserable disabling condition squarely in the hands of the patient.

Over the last decade, Valerie has researched and written this book to help the millions of FMS sufferers all over the world take charge of their condition and heal themselves mentally and physically. This book provides real hope by giving true-life examples as the author courageously tells her story of how she freed herself from the cage of chronic FMS. She has succcessfully regained her health, happiness and prosperity after being bed-ridden for nearly two years and housebound for ten. Now at age 58, Valerie is maintaining her recovery and is fibromyalgia free.

Readers can find Valerie online at: www.thefibrocure.com.